ULTIMATE

Dan
O'Brien's

WORKOUT

ULTIMATE

Dan O'Brien's

WORKOUT

THE GOLD-MEDAL PLAN FOR REACHING YOUR PEAK PERFORMANCE

Dan O'Brien,

OLYMPIC GOLD MEDALIST AND WORLD RECORD HOLDER IN THE DECATHLON

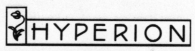

HYPERION

NEW YORK

Library of Congress Cataloging-in-Publication Data
O'Brien, Dan
Dan O'Brien's ultimate workout: the gold-medal plan for reaching your peak performance / Dan O'Brien. — 1st ed.
p. cm.
ISBN 0-7868-8281-6
1. Physical fitness. 2. Physical education and training. 3. O'Brien, Dan. I. Title.
GV481.O28 1997
613.7'11—dc21   97—24500
                                                                      CIP

Designed by Spinning Egg Design Group, Inc.
First Edition
10   9   8   7   6   5   4   3   2   1

I'd like to dedicate this book to the World's Greatest Athlete who exists in all of us.

Acknowledgments

Thank you to Jim Thorpe, whose spirit lives in every multievent athlete in the world.

Thank you to the five existing U.S. Gold Medalists for all of their inspiration:

> Bob Mathias, for doing it first;
>
> Rafer Johnson, for being the most athletic;
>
> Bill Toomey, for making it an art form;
>
> Milt Campbell, for being the most inspirational; and
>
> Bruce Jenner, for his amazing dedication.

I take something from each of you every time I compete.

A special thanks to Rick Sloan, the World's Greatest Coach, for helping me push myself *always*.

A decathlete is only as good as he is coached. Thank you, Brian Tippetts, for just "being Brian."

Thank you Gold Medal Management—Brad Hunt and Janey Miller—for all your caring.

To the entire O'Brien family, I thank you for all of your sacrifices. To Leilani Sang, thank you for sharing all of this with me. Without you, it would not mean as much.

Many thanks also go out to the following individuals who have helped me become the athlete that I am: Jim Reardon, Ron Landeck, Mike Keller, Ron Smith, Larry Hunt, Lee Schroeder, and David Lileks.

Finally, a big thank you to Laura Dayton and Kim Goss for helping me put my thoughts and experiences into words.

TABLE OF CONTENTS

FOREWORD

▲ THE DECATHLON'S STORY

Swedish organizers of the 1912 Stockholm Games were given approval, in 1910, to add several multi-event contests to the Olympic program. The term "tiokamp" or "tikamp" (decathlon) dates to the earliest years of the twentieth century when both Sweden and Denmark borrowed an American event called "All-Around" and experimented with a variety of events. The Swedes devised their own scoring tables and on October 15, 1911, offered the first modern decathlon (with the same events and order but held on a single day) in Goteborg as a practice for the Stockholm Games.

When the decathlon made its Olympic debut the public took notice. The winner became the center of a controversy that would result in the most unfair and regrettable decision ever made by an Olympic sports body. The case lasted for most of the twentieth century.

James Francis Thorpe, part Native American, part Irish, and all athlete, astounded crowds in Stockholm with his record-setting performance in the Olympic decathlon. There were so many entrants that the event had to be spread over three days. Thereafter the decathlon became a two-day event, with the following standard schedule: 100-meter dash, long jump, shot put, high jump, 400-meter race on day one, 110 meter hurdles, discus, pole vault, javelin, and 1500-meter race on day two.

A scoring system based on the current Olympic records in each event was devised by the Swedes to rate the participants and determine the best overall competitor without favoring an athlete who might excel in a few events. The tables have been revised five times (latest revision in 1985) and are still used to determine decathlon standings.

At the Stockholm Olympics in 1912, Jim Thorpe won with well over 8000 points. More impressive was his margin of victory, 688 points ahead of his closest competitor. In the same games, this student from the Carlisle (Penn.) Indian School won the five-event pentathlon, tied for fourth in the high jump, and placed seventh in the long jump. Shortly after the Stockholm Olympics, at an exhibition meet in France for the touring U.S. Olympic Team, Thorpe defeated the new 110-meter hurdle gold medalist Fred Kelly with a time that just missed the existing world record.

Thorpe won the gold as well as the hearts of the people and the acclaim of royalty. He was presented with a pair of gold medals, a jeweled chalice (in the shape of a Viking ship), and a royal bust of King Gustav V of Sweden, who declared, "Sir, you are the greatest athlete in the world." Apocryphally, Jim endearingly responded, "Thanks, King."

Ever since Gustav V's historic statement, every current gold medalist in the decathlon has been known as the "world's greatest athlete."

For Thorpe, that honor would be his for less than a year. In a controversial decision by the Amateur Athletic Union (AAU), Thorpe's records were stricken from the books and he was forced to return his trophies and gold medals. The AAU ruled that he had lost his amateur status by accepting payment for minor league baseball while on vacation several years earlier. The amount was only twenty-five dollars a week and was used to defray Thorpe's living expenses. Thorpe did not realize that his playing would jeopardize his amateur status. Although he later had a long career in baseball and football, he died penniless and medal-less in 1953. Thirty years later fascimile medals were returned to his family, and his name returned to the record books.

In spite of the AAU ruling, sports fans and other athletes who recognized Thorpe's incredible athletic accomplishments never withdrew their admiration. The two athletes to whom Thorpe's gold medals defaulted refused to take physical possession of them. Ferdinand Bie, the Norwegian who placed second in the pentathlon, claimed the gold medal "belonged to Thorpe." Thorpe was indeed the world's greatest athlete and remained the most respected athlete of the twentieth century. When Thorpe died in 1953 the Pennsylvania town of Mauch Chunk changed its name to Jim Thorpe and Jim's body remains buried there to this day.

Thorpe began a tradition of U.S. decathlon success at the Olympic Games. American winners following in Thorpe's footsteps were Harold Osborn in 1924, James Bausch in 1932, Glenn Morris in 1936, Bob Mathias in both 1948 and 1952, Milt Campbell in 1956, Rafer Johnson in 1960, Bill Toomey in 1968, and Bruce Jenner in 1976. But for the next several decades the gold would elude United States decathletes.

The decathlon is an event of economy. The decathlete must be able to weigh each event against the next to determine where too much training in one event may compromise performance in another. Decathletes perform a cost/benefit analysis in every training session and need to be economical with their time and energy.

Many decathletes begin as either hurdlers or sprinters, then are encouraged by their coaches to try the long or high jump. Only after several events are mastered can an athlete even hope to take on the decathlon. A winning decathlete must sacrifice the rewards of excelling in one event for the mastery of all ten.

Since Bruce Jenner's 1976 victory, the U.S. had not won a decathlon gold. Not since Jim Thorpe did the United States have an athlete with the natural potential, will, and attitude to hold onto the title of World's Greatest Athlete. Not until Dan O'Brien came along.

There are parallels between Jim Thorpe and Dan O'Brien that historians cannot ignore. Both were born of mixed races and have Irish surnames. Both came to the Olympics from small schools and small towns. Both experienced major Olympic disappointments. Jim lost his medals while Dan missed a much publicized opportunity to make the 1992 U.S. Olympic Team. Both basked in the adulation of millions. In Dan O'Brien's case, he had the opportunity in 1996 to set the record straight. He faced his moment of truth in Atlanta and prevailed. Today Dan O'Brien carries on the legacy that Jim Thorpe set in motion. Dan O'Brien's story is the future of the decathlon.

—Frank Zarnowski
Emmitsburg, MD
September 1997

ULTIMATE

Dan
O'Brien's

WORKOUT

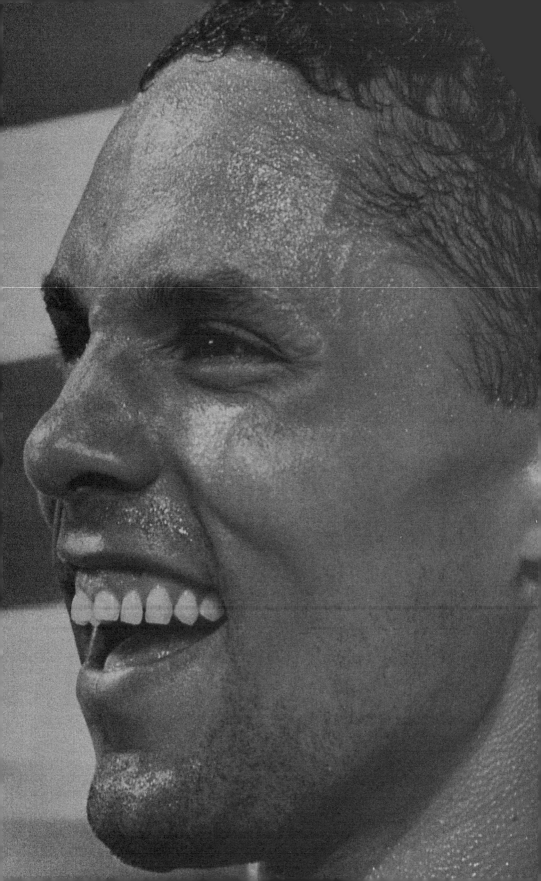

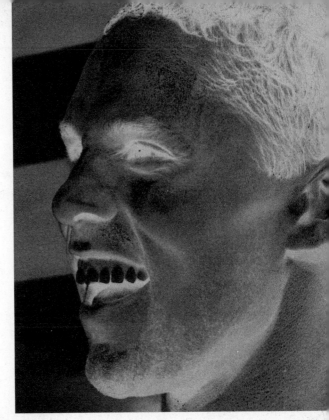

THE
DAN O'BRIEN
STORY

Most babies come into the world crying. Dan O'Brien had better reason than most. Born to a Finnish mother and African-American father in 1966, Dan was immediately put up for adoption. He spent two years in several foster homes. Then Jim and Virginia O'Brien spied this skinny, active toddler and decided to take him into their hearts and home.

At two years old, Dan was given a name. A nice Irish name. He was also given a home in Klamath Falls, Oregon, and would become part of a large family—eight kids in all—six of them adopted and of Asian, Native American and Hispanic origins.

Dan has no memory of the foster homes, but he remembers coming home with the O'Briens and the joy he felt when he first saw his own bedroom. When he talks about his parents and siblings it is with great warmth and genuine love. It was no surprise that the entire O'Brien clan was in the bleachers in Atlanta, often seen trading tickets to get closer to Dan.

Despite the love and support of his family, Dan faced a variety of problems growing up. Dan was hyperactive, and was later diagnosed with attention deficit disorder (ADD). School was tough for Dan, and running off excess energy was his way of coping. The O'Briens tell stories about how Dan was running when other children his age were waddling. When he played Little League baseball, people would come just to see him race around the bases. Dan was born to run.

One of the things Dan doesn't run from is his past. "There are certain issues that you deal with as an adopted child," he says. "There are holes in my past, and as a teenager, I struggled with my identity. I used to call myself a chameleon because I could fit in almost anywhere. I'd hang out with various groups of people in school, always trying to find where I belonged. Relating to my African-American identity was tough. Raised by Caucasian parents, I really knew nothing about being black."

At times in his life Dan has thought about seeking the identities of his birth parents, but he shakes his head about such a search today. "I've got a family, and I just don't think it's a big thing."

Dan has faced other difficult issues. A star high school athlete in track, baseball and basketball, he was recruited by the University of Idaho on a full track scholarship. Working with coach Mike Keller, Dan found himself on the brink of a promising sports career. Unfortunately, academics were not his strong point, and though he was managing his ADD effectively, Dan preferred running and jumping and partying. And that's exactly what he did, until his grades fell so low he lost his scholarship.

"I looked at my life and realized things had to change. That was one of the first times I connected with the fact that an athlete can't get along on raw talent alone. I realized that I was going to have to make some sacrifices and put my nose to the grindstone."

Dan decided he wanted to be an athlete instead of a dropout, and coach Keller was there to work with him. Dan enrolled in a junior college, stopped partying, and began training seriously.

"I didn't set out to be a decathlete, but my speed gave me a natural edge. I was outscoring everyone, without putting in much effort," says Dan about his 1988 decision to pursue the decathlon. "As I looked at the opportunities and where I held the strongest advantage, the decathlon just kept coming up as the best choice. It is also the ultimate challenge, and the athlete in me found that irresistible. Of course, the fact that its winner is the World's Greatest Athlete also had a strong appeal for me. I decided that was what I wanted to become."

In 1991, Dan became the Decathlon World Champion.

Until a few years ago, most people couldn't even name the ten events that comprise the decathlon, or knew who held the world record. Things changed in 1992 when Reebok aired the first ad of its "Dan and Dave" advertising campaign on Super Bowl Sunday. The campaign played on the rivalry between two of America's best decathletes as they prepared for the Olympics in Barcelona. Dan and fellow decathlete Dave Johnson became overnight celebrities.

"I was recognized everywhere I went," remembers Dan. "We didn't get paid much for it, but the campaign certainly put us in the spotlight. I can't say I didn't enjoy it—to the contrary, it was great."

Great, for a time. During the Olympic trials the Reebok publicity machine made certain that all eyes were focused on Dan and Dave. For the only time in his life, none of Dan's attempts at the pole vault succeeded. That infamous "no-heighter" cost him his place on the Olympic team. He was now the most famous failure in sports, branded by the media as soft-headed and fainthearted.

For most of the world, that was where the Dan O'Brien story ended. That is, until he handily won the gold medal at the 1996 Atlanta Games. For Dan O'Brien, the no-heighter was simply another issue to put behind him, which he did in a very definitve way.

At the 1992 Barcelona Olympics, Dan cheered the athletes with genuine enthusiasm, even though he was sidelined rather than out on the field where he belonged. "It was crushing for me. It was unbelievably hard," he admits. But to the audience who listened to his track and field commentary on NBC, there wasn't a trace of bitterness. His affable personality comes through as clearly in the face of personal disaster as it does when Dan achieves personal triumph.

After Barcelona, Dan went back to training and competed in the decathlon event in Talence, France, in 1992. There he set a new world record—8,891 points, a record that was still standing when Dan went to Atlanta in 1996. Dan went on to win two more world championships before the 1996 Olympic trials rolled around. And once again, America's eyes were trained on Dan O'Brien as he faced the pole vault.

The media focused on Dan's vault, but the truth was that Dan had long ago come to terms with the 1992 fiasco.

"I don't know that I'll ever know exactly what went wrong that day," says Dan. "I do know that as an athlete I've learned to prepare myself for any eventuality, to train for each event as hard as I possibly can, to come in as prepared mentally and physically as possible.

"For me, the pole vault wasn't an issue. Getting on the team wasn't an issue—I knew I was prepared for the gold; the trials were just a step on the way."

Dan cleared his first vault and went on to clear over 17 feet. Then he set a personal best in the javelin with 214 feet, giving him the best decathlon score ever through nine events. As he prepared for the 1500 meters, the final event of the decathlon and Dan's least favorite, he was close to breaking his own world record. That didn't happen this time, but Dan gained his spot on the Atlanta Olympic team and was on his way to erasing the lingering taint of the 1992 no-heighter from his reputation.

Dan's superior conditioning was as much the result of his more mature, stable attitude as it was the excellent coaching he'd been receiving during the past six years from Rick Sloan. Under Sloan's tutelage, Dan went from being an athlete who needed to be told what to do to an athlete who not only knew what to do, but who took total joy in doing it. Dan had truly become the ultimate athlete.

In Atlanta, Dan became the first American to win the decathlon since Bruce Jenner in 1976. His only disappointment was that, in the process, he did not break his own world record. That is something he's working on.

Atlanta wasn't Dan's best decathlon pointwise, but it was his vindication. The first day of decathlon ended with Dan clearly out in front of his closest competitor. The second day began on a wet and sloppy 110-meter track. Dan crossed the finish line for the 110-meter hurdles behind Germany's Frank Busemann and held onto an overall lead of just 71 points. Next, Dan spun the discus to a distance just behind Belorussian Eduard Hamalainen to hold onto a lead of 142. In the following event, Dan faced the pole vault pit, where he played it conservatively and cleared 16 feet, 5 inches, the same height as Hamalainen, to remain 142 points up. The points were jockeyed throughout the two-day event, but O'Brien held his lead. Before a crowd of nearly eighty-three-thousand screaming fans, Dan came up for his final throw of the javelin. Dan raised his spear, then ran, skipped and over-handed his throw to the roar of the crowd—a roar that grew deafening as the missile continued to arc through the air. It planted itself at a personal best of 219 feet, 6 inches—two inches farther than the throw of Dan's closest rival.

The final event of the day, the 1500 meters, has always been Dan's toughest. After two days of competition and nine events, Dan knew he needed to stay within 32 seconds of Busemann to capture the gold. The camera captured Dan's intensity—the gritted teeth, the grimace as the final gun went off. In a dramatic finish in front of a standing audience, Dan crossed the finish line just 14.48 seconds behind his challenger and into the history books.

For many years it seemed that Dan would forever be plagued by his "eleventh event"—his failures. Now it seems those are permanently behind him. He has earned a respected place in sports history. He wears the badge of the World's Greatest Athlete proudly. He doesn't hide from his past, but uses it to help other young athletes overcome the pitfalls that face every athlete today.

Dan has been extremely active in youth programs. He uses his own educational and social battles to help at-risk students improve their academic performance. He is presently involved in a poster program aimed predominantly at middle school students. The program encourages students to write to Dan and share their own stories. In return, Dan sends them a personal letter, two trading cards and a one-page biography. He is involved in a charity golf tournament to benefit children's educational groups.

Dan is also sharing his training knowledge with others to help people achieve a higher level of fitness and health. One big step toward that end is this book.

"The decathlon is the ultimate athletic event. It is the measuring stick for athletic achievement. A marathon runner may be great at running long distances, but he may not be healthy. A baseball player may have great hand-eye coordination, but he may not be fit. A football player may be strong, but he might not live past fifty. On the other hand, a decathlete is fast, coordinated, strong and—most of all—fit and healthy."

This book won't teach you how to win a gold medal, but it may inspire you to try. It brings together Dan's unique perspectives on the elements of total fitness. Different from other programs predicated on losing weight or building bulging biceps, this program is about achieving fitness as a by-product of enhanced athletic performance. By following Dan's unique progam, you will find yourself better equipped for performance, whether your sport is the decathlon, bowling, golf, football or aerobic dance. His ultimate program tells you how to get in the best shape of your life, for sports, vitality and longevity. It's a balanced program based on sound principles and some cutting-edge information that only the World's Greatest Athlete can provide.

Expect to work hard when you follow Dan's program. Expect the results to be worth the effort.

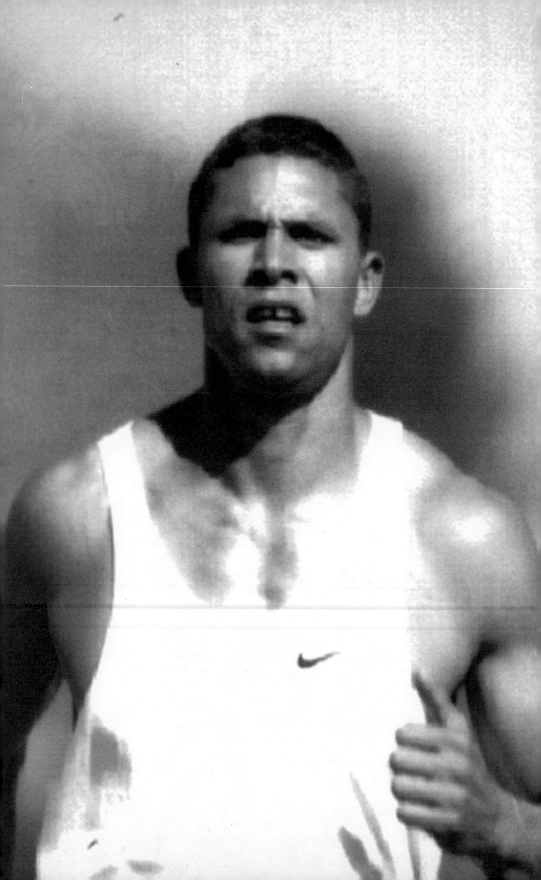

COMPONENTS

OF TOTAL

FITNESS

I was born athletic. My mom loves to tell people that even as a toddler I'd tuck in my chin, dig in my toes and take off like a bullet with my skinny arms pumping the air. I can remember discovering the sheer joy of running on the playgrounds and fields of my hometown, Klamath Falls, Oregon. I still enjoy running, but it's a bit more complex now. I've made the transition from being athletic to being an athlete.

If you want to pursue a professional career in sports, it's an initial distinction to understand. I was naturally talented, but learning to focus and harness my athletic abilities was absolutely essential to learning how to win. Succeeding as an athlete today means you've got to tackle every challenge with the attitude that you're going to win; you've got to *want* to win, and then you've got to win.

I remember standing in the pouring rain behind the blocks at my first World Championships in Tokyo. A lot of the other athletes were complaining about the bad conditions; you could see the distraction in their body language. I looked up and let the rain hit me in the face. I wasn't afraid of it. I thought, It's raining today, but somebody still has to win, and it's going to be me. I also knew if I didn't win, I'd have to go back and find a way to win. I've always been able to find a way to challenge myself, and that's one of the most important things that has helped me succeed.

However, all the attitude in the world isn't going to get you over your first hurdle if you don't have a good conditioning program. Even if you run for a few years on good genes and adrenaline, once you get serious—whether about one specific sport or ten—your general conditioning is of paramount importance. Keeping yourself focused is a critical factor in your success as an athlete, but seeing the broad picture is essential to achieving maximum performance from your body. Of course, a balanced program is the key to optimum results, and nobody knows that better than a decathlete. If I spent all my time working on running speed, I'd compromise my strength and jumping ability. If I spent all my time working on javelin, my endurance and running speed would suffer. If I spent all my time on the decathlete events and neglected the warm-ups, cooldowns, massages, stretching and weight work, I wouldn't have the gold medal today.

Anyone seriously involved in a sport, whether for fun or competition, risks developing muscle imbalances if he or she doesn't follow a balanced training program. These imbalances often lead to postural problems that can create or aggravate many orthopedic conditions (particularly in the lower back) and, in the long run, have a devastating effect on your general health. Preventing injury is an important element of my program, but the truth is a solid and well-balanced conditioning regimen also will help you perform better at a specific sport—or, as in my case, ten of them.

Many athletes use crosstraining to effectively combat the negative effects of sport-specific training and to prevent muscle imbalances. Crosstraining also adds variety to an athlete's regimen—variety that will continually encourage the body to improve and keep enthusiasm high.

Crosstraining has become a popular term that many people use, not really knowing what it means. There are actually two basic types of crosstraining: concurrent and complementary. Concurrent crosstraining occurs when an athlete uses another sport to *enhance* performance in his or her primary sport. Examples of this type of crosstraining include basketball and volleyball, soccer and field hockey, rowing and kayaking, and ice skating and in-line skating. Complementary crosstraining occurs when an athlete uses another sport to *balance* the training of the primary sport. Examples of this type of crosstraining include running and rowing, cycling and handball, swimming and soccer.

Decathlon Crosstraining Conditioning Groups			
Speed	**Strength**	**Jumping**	**Endurance**
100 meter sprint	discus	high jump	400 meters
hurdles	shot put	long jump	1500 meters
	javelin	pole vault	

As a decathlete, it's safe to say I'm the ultimate crosstrainer, using both concurrent and complementary crosstraining. I split my event training over two days, as in an actual decathlon. On the first day, I practice the 100 meters, long jump, shot put, high jump, and the 400 meters. On the second day, I practice the high hurdles, discus, pole vault, javelin, and the 1500. I usually train the events twice a week. Though I practice the ultimate crosstraining mix, I still perform general conditioning exercises three days a week—every week, even during the few weeks out of the year that I don't do specific work. This is all in addition to my stretching and endurance work.

Sport-specific training, even in a healthy crosstraining mix, can never totally replace general conditioning. I've been blessed with a relatively injury-free career because I've always placed a high priority on general conditioning. The sport work is fun and rewarding because you always have benchmarks—a time to beat, a distance to top—but general conditioning needs to be approached differently, more like a lifestyle than an activity. You should get into the habit of a regular program of exercise, just as you get up every morning and go through a ritual of showering, combing your hair and getting dressed. In the same way that you take an hour or so out of every day to have lunch, you need to devote time on a consistent basis to make certain your body is properly conditioned.

This book shows you the ultimate training routine. The workout and fitness advice I'm offering you is based on my own career and training, as well as information gleaned from coaches and other athletes over the years. Reading this book may not win you a gold medal, but it will give you some of the tools you need to win. Though I'll share with you some of my experiences in winning the gold, this isn't a book about the Olympics, or even the decathlon. This is a book about the ultimate workout.

I'm not going to tell you that you can get great abs in three weeks or that you'll learn to throw the javelin by page 89. I will, however, give you workout and exercise advice to make you healthier, stronger, faster, and more agile, athletic, and coordinated. My intent is to give you the ultimate program, one that deals with all the components of total fitness. Here are the four components of my program:

▲ **Agility/Flexibility Development**

▲ **Strength Training**

▲ **Ballistic Strength Training**

▲ **Energy Training**

Each of these components improves basic *physical* fitness; and when performed in conjunction with the others, will dramatically improve the specific *athletic fitness* necessary for peak sport performance. How and to what degree each of these components fits into your weekly schedule is dependent upon your goals and present conditioning level. If you're a competitive athlete, you might consider this chapter an off-season training guide. As your competitive season nears, you would logically need to cut back on some of these drills to accommodate sport-specific work to peak for competition. If you're a weekend warrior, I suggest following a program that contains each of these elements of fitness on a consistent basis, year in and year out. Whether that is two times a week or five times a week is up to you.

My program is focused on an athletic vantage point rather than concentrating on weight loss or physique development. If you follow this program, your body weight will probably drop by a few pounds and you will have more control over your weight. However, the results you will achieve will be most apparent in your performance. If you ski, you'll ski longer and harder. If volleyball is your game, you'll serve stronger and with more accuracy. If you bowl, you'll play with more ease and control. Your heart will be healthier, your muscles stronger, and your coordination better.

▲ THE ULTIMATE SPORT

I will also teach you about the decathlon. I'll share some of my favorite moments and give you pointers for individual events. One of my goals is to help the decathlon grow in participation. I hope this book inspires more talented athletes to tackle my sport. And, I *dream* that hundreds of young athletes will set goals of becoming the World's Greatest Athlete.

The "money sports"—basketball, football, baseball— attract a majority of today's most talented athletes. I sometimes wonder what the decathlon totals would be if athletes like Bo Jackson chose to participate.

The decathlon is a pure sport. Its competitors are the healthiest of all athletes because they must master every component of fitness—speed, endurance, strength, and coordination. It requires total commitment and dedication. It is truly the measuring stick of human athletic potential: How high can we jump, how far can we jump, how fast can we run, how far can we run, how far can we throw?

To compete effectively in any sport, you have to train effectively. To do so requires goals, and then a plan to reach those goals. A long-range goal should be set as high as your imagination allows. For me, it was simple: I wanted to be the World's Greatest Athlete. I wanted to set the world record. I wanted to win a gold medal. I still want to reach a total of 9,000 points, although 9,125 (the goal I wrote on my cap in Atlanta) would be even better. I want a total that will stand for many years to come.

Goal setting is part of the ultimate workout because, without it, your program will fail. Before you go any further, stop and assess your personal goals. Once you've identified a long-term goal, you must get to work on the incremental steps that will allow you to accomplish it. These interim steps should be your weekly, biweekly or monthly benchmarks. You need to chronicle your training and look for constant improvements. You want to move that carrot just a few inches further from your grasp. Then, when you've reached a certain level, you want to continue to track your performance to make certain you don't backslide.

The ultimate training program must address all the components of fitness, and then some. Faced with so many physical challenges, a successful athlete must have total self-control. You must learn to be totally in control of your performance. As you complete each incremental task, as you monitor and make a checklist so that every aspect of your training has been attended to, your confidence will increase.

I'm a full-time athlete. I train at least ten months out of the year, several hours a day, six days a week. During the months I take off, my training is reduced to three days a week. I never stop training, nor will I—until I retire with a nine-thousand-point total.

Making this kind of commitment to a sport requires that you set incremental goals to keep you focused and seeing results. Results are what will keep you reaching for the next step. Whether you pursue a serious career in sports or just want to achieve your personal best and live life to its fullest, small goals are what will get you there.

This program addresses the four crucial components of ultimate fitness. Treat each one separately, and schedule them into your life based on your goals, your present level of fitness, your lifestyle, and your available time. But fit them in—then begin taking the tiny steps that will inch you ever closer to better health and longevity.

COMPONENT ONE
▲ AGILITY/FLEXIBILITY DEVELOPMENT

Two things come to mind when aspiring athletes think of athletic training—firstly, maximizing the results from every workout or drill, and secondly, injury prevention. When *world-class* athletes think of training, what comes to mind first is injury prevention.

I love sports of all kinds, and there is not a sport I can't perform at least at average level, including tennis, basketball, snow skiing, waterskiing, table tennis, badminton, bowling, volleyball, and golf. I enjoyed them all, until I realized I was capable of achieving a world record. Then sports for pleasure presented a risk I couldn't afford to take. I've avoided staircases for fear of twisting an ankle, and I avoid night running. You might think the staircase behavior borders on the extreme, but the level of performance asked of today's world-class athletes is extreme. As the saying goes, "You must rise to meet the challenge."

WARMING UP

An injury is every serious athlete's worst nightmare. Injuries are also cumulative in nature, and an accumulation is to be avoided at all costs. It pains me to see an athlete like Jackie Joyner-Kersee sidelined because of injuries, or even my Reebok rival Dave Johnson. Both Jackie and Dave began their professional athletic careers at much younger ages than I (I wasn't a serious contender until I was in my twenties). Starting late has helped to minimize my injuries. Additionally, I am extremely keen on utilizing every means of injury prevention available.

At the top of my list are proper warm-ups and cooldowns. I am a firm believer in regular body work—it is absolutely essential to the longevity of any athlete to keep the skeletal muscles flexible and resilient through regular stretching and massage.

I begin every workout with a warm-up. One of the purposes of a warm-up is to raise your overall body temperature, especially in the muscles. Research has shown that increasing body temperature improves performance by enabling the muscles to contract faster and more intensely. Stretching also helps prevent injury by increasing range of motion. A warm-up can be accomplished in a variety of ways, but I prefer to begin with stretching, followed by a short jog. On hurdling days, I do additional hamstring and calf stretches during my warm-up. On javelin days I add javelin-specific stretches.

The best stretching is called *passive*, meaning that you use a partner (or a towel or rope) to increase the depth of a stretch. In passive stretching, the muscles surrounding the area being stretched are not involved in generating the stretching force so you can relax more completely and stretch further. I move into a stretch slowly, then hold it for thirty to forty-five seconds. On most training days I perform all the stretches demonstrated here, but each day's mood and regimen dictates certain revisions in my routine. The bottom line is to be sure to properly stretch the muscles to be worked on a given day. On my off days, I use a slightly modified routine.

A proper cooldown consists of low-intensity exercises to lower the body temperature and respiration (walking is ideal) and includes additional essential stretching movements. Stretching after a workout helps remove the muscle tension that develops during exercise. A cooldown stretch is generally performed more slowly, allowing the tension to flow out of the muscle so that it can relax to its fullest. I use many of the same stretches in the cooldown that I used in the warm-up, paying particular attention to stretching the muscles I've just worked.

Stretching not only prepares a muscle for work and relaxes a muscle after work, but also contributes to an athlete's overall agility and coordination. Even in weight training I try to achieve a full range of motion. Partial movements and cheating techniques are the stuff that make high school boys seem macho, but they have no place in a serious athlete's routine.

The benefits of stretching are many; a regular program can help you avoid muscle strains and soreness, improve your posture, relax tense muscles, and relieve and even resolve back pain. It feels good, and its benefits can be achieved in just a few minutes a day. You can stretch at home, even at work. In fact, you can stretch pretty much anytime and anywhere.

Stretching develops self-discipline and helps you achieve a mind-muscle relationship. It is important for athletes to give themselves totally to the task at hand, which means putting one hundred percent of your concentration and involvement into stretching sessions. You need to actually feel your muscle, to become familiar with the feeling of tension, and to learn how to eliminate it. Accomplishing ultimate muscle control is necessary for me because of the diversity of decathlon events. When I see photos of myself preparing for the javelin, I can see the flexion in my upper-body muscles—my delts are striated and my pecs full. Yet in photos of my track events, my upper body muscles seem to relax and I focus my energy into my lower body, which translates to a visible delineation of the muscles in my legs. Achieving this type of muscle selectivity comes partly from the quiet times I spend stretching and learning to focus my concentration on specific muscle groups.

There are a few conditions under which you shouldn't stretch; for example, you shouldn't stretch the area around a bone that's been recently fractured, or an area that has been recently sprained or strained. There are also certain vascular problems and skin diseases for which stretching may be considered harmful. If you have a question, you should always consult an expert.

One of the current theories about stretching is that it is better to perform the majority of your passive stretching after a workout, or as a workout in itself. It's believed that passive stretching may prevent you from achieving a high level of muscular contractions if it is performed immediately before explosive activities such as the shot put. This theory would not apply to long-distance running.

Also, you should ideally stretch in loose, comfortable clothing. A firm, nonskid mat is great, and the area should be quiet so you can concentrate.

◆DAN'S STRETCHES

ADDUCTORS

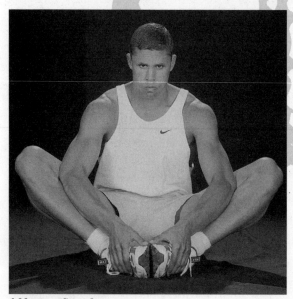

Adductors Stretch

Sit upright on the floor. Bend your knees and pull your feet as close to your hips as possible; your feet should be touching each other. Keeping your chest up and back flat, perform the stretch by pressing your knees downward as far as is comfortable with your elbows. Hold, and then return to the starting position.

DAN'S TIPS: If you find it difficult to keep your back straight during this stretch, perform it with your back against a wall.

ADDUCTORS

Stand and point your toes slightly out to the sides. Bend forward from the waist slightly, lower your hips and extend your left leg (also known in this stretch as the support leg) directly out to the side. When your left thigh is parallel to the floor, increase the stretch on the inside of the left thigh by pushing your hips down

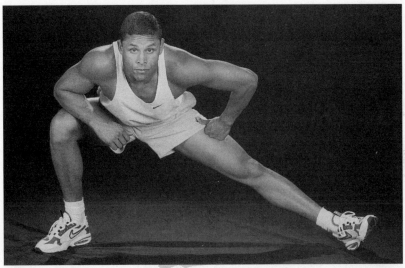

Adductors Stretch

and towards the left foot, keeping the support knee in alignment with the foot. Straighten your legs to return to the start, then repeat for the other side.

DAN'S TIPS: If you have trouble maintaining your balance when you first attempt this stretch, place a chair or other sturdy object in front of you and hold on to it for support.

Adductors Stretch

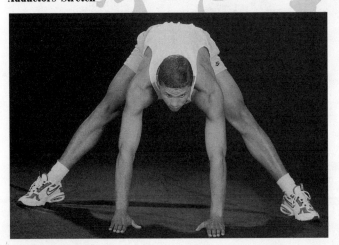

ADDUCTORS

Stand and spread your legs about four feet apart. Keeping your legs straight but not hyperextended, lean forward from the waist as far

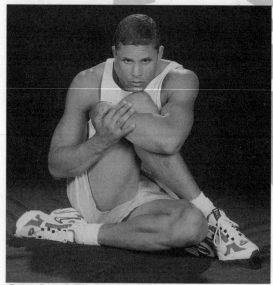

as possible without rounding your back. Increase the stretch by moving your feet further apart.

DAN'S TIPS: If you cannot reach the floor without round- ing your back when you first perform this stretch, place a chair in front of you for balance and bend only as far as good technique allows.

Buttock and Hip Stretch (1)

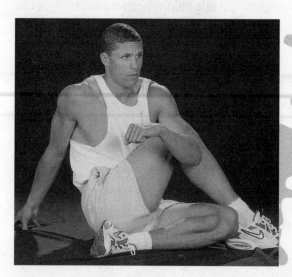

BUTTOCKS AND HIPS

This is a two-part stretch. Sit upright on the floor and cross your right leg over your left.

Buttock and Hip Stretch (2)

Keeping your back flat, grasp your right leg with both hands and lean forward.

For the second part of this stretch, place your right arm behind your back and the upper part of your left arm behind your right leg. Using your left arm for leverage, twist your waist to the left.

Return to the start and repeat for the other side.

DAN'S TIPS: For maximum effectiveness, you must keep your torso as erect as possible as you perform both parts of this stretch.

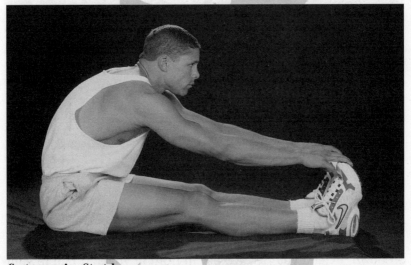

Gastrocnemius Stretch

GASTROCNEMIUS

Sit down on the floor and extend your legs in front of you, knees straight and feet together. Lean forward from the waist, bend your knees, and grasp the fronts of your feet. Perform the stretch by bending forward from the hips.

DAN'S TIPS: You can also perform this stretch by placing a towel around your feet and pulling on the towel rather than leaning forward. This will enable you to perform the stretch without having to round your back excessively.

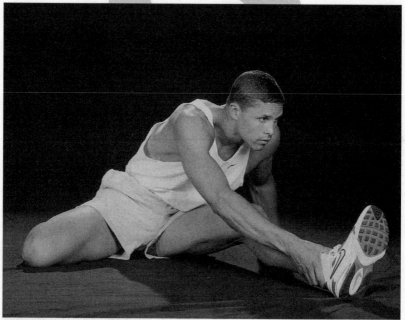

Hamstrings Stretch

HAMSTRINGS

Sit down, extend your left leg out in front of you and pull in your right leg under and back behind you, as close to your hip as possible. Place your hands together on your left knee. Without rounding your back, lean forward as far as comfortable, hold, and then return to the start. Repeat for the other leg.

DAN'S TIPS: If you feel pain in your knees while performing this exercise, pull in your trailing leg so that your right foot touches the inside of your thigh.

HIP FLEXORS

From a standing position, place your hands on your hips and point your toes straight ahead. Keeping your torso upright, step backward and bend your knees until your rear knee touches the floor (or as far as comfortable). Keeping the forward knee perpendicular to the floor, push your hips down and forward to increase the stretch. Return to the start by stepping forward with the rear leg, then repeat the stretch for the other side.

DAN'S TIPS: If you have trouble balancing in the deep lunge position of this stretch, place your hands on your forward knee.

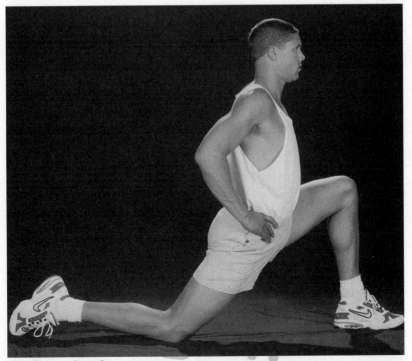

Hip Flexors Stretch

HIPS AND QUADRICEPS

This is a two-part stretch. Sit upright on the floor. Bend your left knee outward and your right knee inward so that your left foot

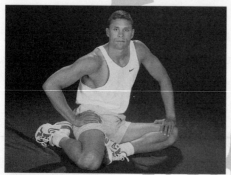

Hips and Quadriceps Stretch (1)

touches the outside of your right thigh and your right heel touches your right hip. From this starting position, bend forward from the waist with your arms extended in front of you. Lower your head and chest as far as comfortable, then return to the start.

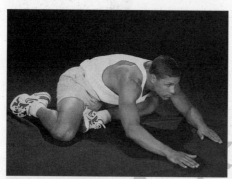

Hips and Quadriceps Stretch (2)

For the second part of this stretch, simply lean back as far as comfortable, hold, then return to the start.

DAN'S TIPS: To compensate for poor flexibility, some individuals will lift their hips as they bend from the waist. Be aware of this tendency, and only stretch as far as is comfortable.

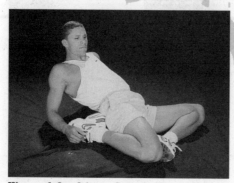

Hips and Quadriceps Stretch (3)

LOWER BACK

Sit down on the floor and extend your legs in front of you, knees straight and feet together. Extend your arms out to your sides. Lie back and, while keeping your legs straight, bring your feet up and behind your head as far as you can while keeping your shoulder blades in contact with the floor—if you feel any pressure on your neck, you're performing it incorrectly.

DAN'S TIPS: As you become more flexible, bring your arms back and try to grab your toes. This will stretch your gastrocnemius and, to a lesser extent, your hamstrings.

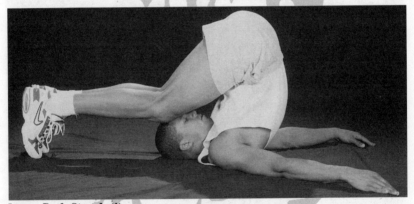

Lower Back Stretch (1)

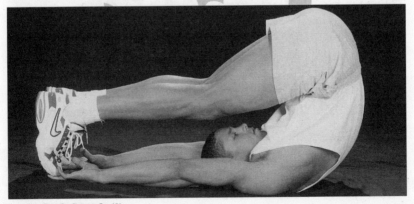

Lower Back Stretch (2)

SHOULDERS

Lie on your right side. Place your left arm in front of you for balance and your right arm back behind you, palm down, as shown. Using the left arm for support, lower your right shoulder as far as possible. Repeat for the other side.

DAN'S TIPS: If this exercise is too intense, try performing it from a standing position against a wall until your flexibility improves.

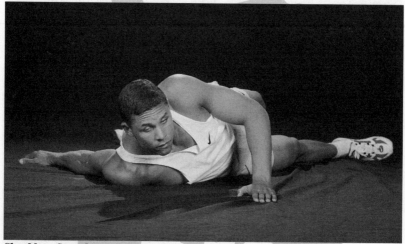

Shoulders Stretch

SHOULDER ROTATION

Grasp a stick, palms down, and spread your hands as far apart as possible. Keeping your arms straight, lift the stick above and then behind you in one continuous motion as far as you can. Increase the difficulty of this stretch by moving your hands closer together.

DAN'S TIPS: If this exercise bothers your wrists, try performing it by holding the stick between your thumb and index finger. This variation will alter the position of your hand so that there is less stretch on the wrists. Some people may have trouble bringing the bar behind their necks—do so only as far as you can.

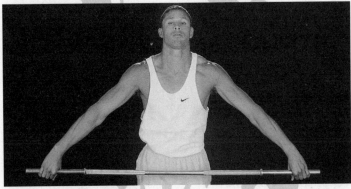

Shoulder Rotation Stretch (1)

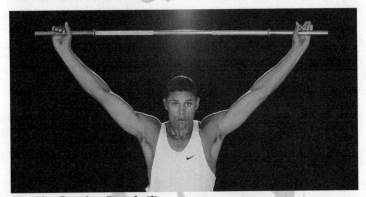

Shoulder Rotation Stretch (2)

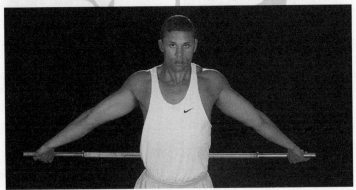

Shoulder Rotation Stretch (3)

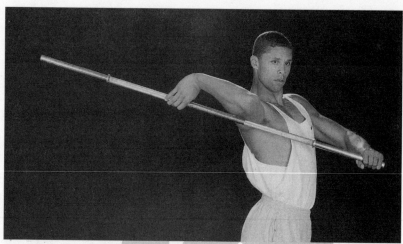

Shoulder External Rotation Stretch

SHOULDER EXTERNAL ROTATION

Grasp one end of a stick with your right hand so that the other end of the stick is resting on the back of your lower right arm. Grasp this end of the stick with the left hand. Begin the stretch by lifting up on the end of the stick with your left hand so that your right arm externally rotates. Repeat for the other arm.

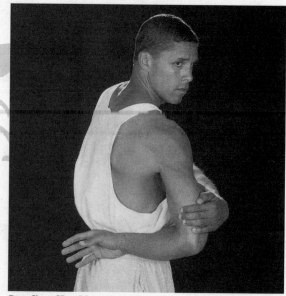

DAN'S TIPS: This exercise can also be per-formed seated.

Standing Shoulders Stretch

STANDING SHOULDERS

From a standing position, bend your right arm inward to 45 degrees over your shoulders and behind your back as shown. Your palm should be facing away from the body. Increase the stretch by using your other hand to push your elbow down further. Repeat for the other side.

DAN'S TIPS: You can also make the exercise more difficult by moving your hand further up your back.

SOLEUS

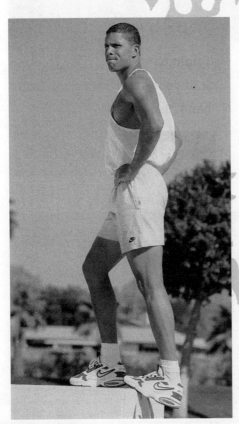

Soleus Stretch

Stand on the edge of a step or platform. Move one foot behind the other so that the ball of the foot is on the edge of the step and your heel extends beyond the edge. Bend your rear leg slightly. Begin the stretch by pressing the near heel down as far as is comfortable. Repeat for the other leg.

DAN'S TIPS: By performing this exercise with the knee straight, you can also stretch the gastrocnemius calf muscle.

TORSO

From a standing position, place a stick on your shoulders behind your neck. Stand and spread your legs to shoulder width and bend your knees slightly. Keeping your shoulder in line with the stick, rotate your waist and hips to the left, back to center, and then to the right.

DAN'S TIPS: To get a greater stretch of the obliques, perform this exercise seated.

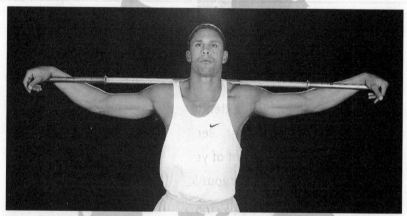

Torso Stretch (1)

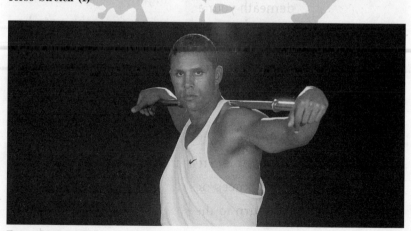

Torso Stretch (2)

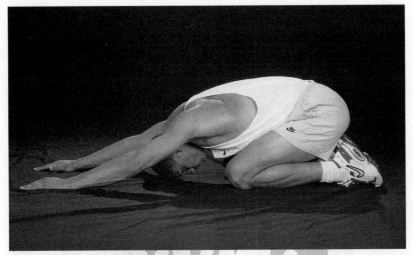

Upper Back and Shins Stretch

UPPER BACK AND SHINS

Kneel down with your feet extended so that the tops of your feet are in contact with the floor. Bend forward from the waist and extend your arms out in front of you, palms down. Continue leaning forward, trying to touch your head to the floor.

DAN'S TIPS: If this stretch is too intense for your shins, place a rolled-up towel underneath your ankles.

◆ PARTNER-ASSISTED STRETCHES

ADDUCTORS

Sit upright on the floor. Bend your knees and pull your feet as close to your hips as possible. From this starting position, have your partner press your knees downward as far as is comfortable, hold, and then return to the start.

DAN'S TIPS: One of the most common technique faults in this stretch is rounding your back. This can be prevented by concentrating on lifting your chest up as you stretch.

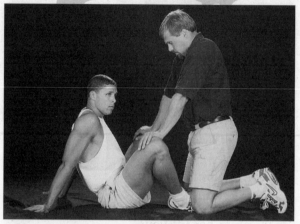

Partner-Assissted Adductors Stretch (1)

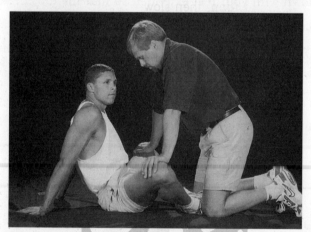

Partner-Assissted Adductors Stretch (2)

BUTTOCKS AND LOWER BACK

Lie face up and bend one leg so that the lower leg is perpendicular to the floor. Have a partner kneel beside you, and have him or her

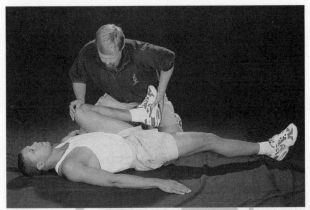

Partner-Assisted Buttocks and Lower Back Stretch

grasp one ankle and position himself as shown. His or her other leg stabilizes the non-exercising leg. While your partner stabilizes your free leg, have him or her lift your knee up as far as comfortable, hold at the top position, then slowly lower the leg. Repeat for the other side.

DAN'S TIPS: Do not allow the hips to raise off the floor as you perform this exercise.

CHEST AND SHOULDERS

Sit upright, crossing your ankles in front of you. Have a partner stand behind you and grasp your arms at the elbows, allowing your upper and lower arms to form

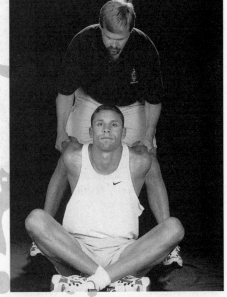

**Partner-Assisted
Chest and Shoulders Stretch**

forty-five-degree angles. Keeping your chest up and shoulders back, have your partner lift your upper arms until they are parallel to the floor, then pull them together to complete the stretch.

DAN'S TIPS: Keep your shoulders down and relaxed as you are being stretched—let your partner do all the work.

CHEST, SHOULDERS, AND ARMS

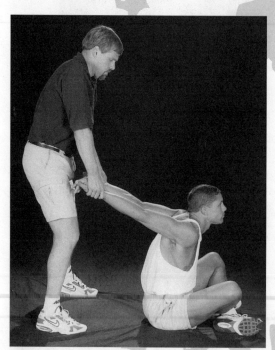

Partner-Assisted Chest, Shoulders, and Arms Stretch

Sit upright, crossing your ankles in front of you. Have a partner stand behind you and grasp your arms at the wrists. Your palms should be turned down. Keeping your chest up and shoulders back, have your partner lift your arms until they are slightly above parallel to the floor, then pull them together to complete the stretch.

DAN'S TIPS: Keep your shoulders down and relaxed as you are being stretched—let your partner do all the work.

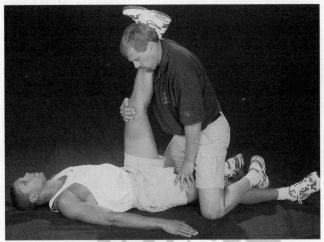

Partner-Assisted Hamstring Stretch

HAMSTRINGS

Lie face up and with both legs extended in front of you. Have a partner kneel beside you, and have him or her grasp one ankle as you rest your lower leg on his shoulder while anchoring your other leg against one of his lower legs. Have your partner lift your knee up and back as far as comfortable, hold at the top position, then slowly lower the leg. Repeat for the other side.

DAN'S TIPS: This exercise must be performed cautiously, as it doesn't require much movement to achieve maximum stretch.

QUADRICEPS I

Lie face down and bend one leg so that the lower leg is perpendicular to the floor. Have a partner kneel beside you and place one hand under your bent knee and the other on your lower back or glutes. While your partner stabilizes your lower back, have him or

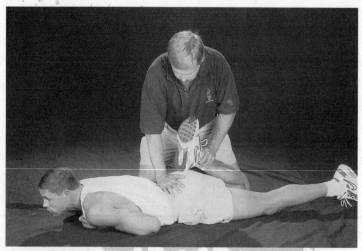

Partner-Assisted Quadriceps I Stretch

her lift your knee up as far as comfortable, hold at the top position, then slowly lower the leg. Repeat for the other side.

DAN'S TIPS: This exercise must be performed cautiously, as it doesn't require much movement to achieve maximum stretch.

QUADRICEPS II

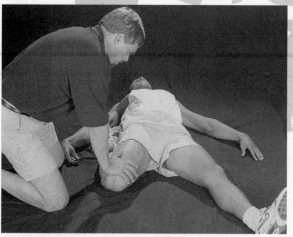

Partner-Assisted Quadriceps II Stretch

Sit down, place your left foot out in front of you and pull in your right leg under and back behind you, as close to your hips as possible. Place your hands together on your left knee. From this position, lean as far back as comfortable, keeping your front knee down. Now have your partner press down on the knee to increase the stretch. Return to the start and repeat for the other leg.

DAN'S TIPS: People often try to cheat on this stretch by arching their backs. Hold your abdominals in while performing this exercise and try to press your lower back to the floor.

STANDING SHOULDERS

This exercise requires a standing position and is best performed with a partner. Have a partner grasp your right arm, palm down, with his or her right hand and place the other hand under your elbow. Begin the exercise by turning away from your partner and rotating your hand up (external rotation). Increase the stretch by increasing the amount you turn.

DAN'S TIPS: If a partner is not available, use a cable apparatus or rope set about shoulder height.

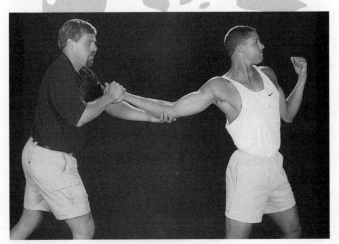

Partner-Assisted Standing Shoulders Stretch

◆ DYNAMIC STRETCHES

Dynamic stretches improve the coordination, strength, and elasticity of your muscles. These are performed before sprinting and jumping and after weight training. Dynamic stretching and ballistic stretching are not the same. With ballistic stretching you use momentum, rather than muscular control, to increase your range of motion. With dynamic stretching you are always in control throughout the entire range of motion—there are no bouncing or jerking movements.

As a general rule, you should perform dynamic stretches for sets of at least ten repetitions, with rests of about one minute between sets of the same exercise. Begin each movement slowly, gradually increasing the speed and the range of motion of each exercise.

FREE LEG SWINGS—FRONTAL

Stand so that you can hold on to a sturdy object as shown. Swing the leg furthest from your support as shown, balancing on the ball of your other foot. Complete all the reps for one leg before facing the other direction and working the other leg.

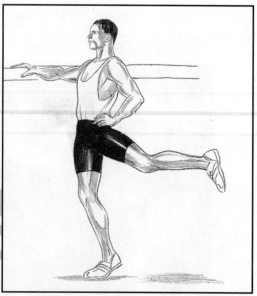

Free Leg Swings—Frontal Stretch (1)

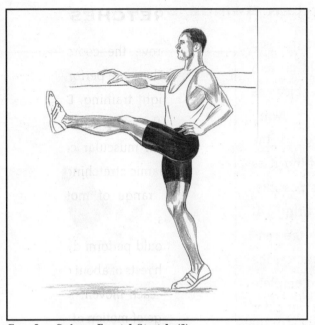

Free Leg Swings—Frontal Stretch (2)

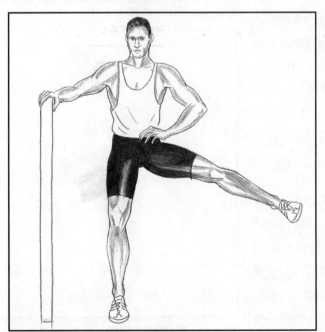

Free Leg Swings—Sagittal Stretch

FREE LEG SWINGS—SAGITTAL

Stand so that you can hold on to a sturdy object as shown. Swing one leg to the side, lifting it as high as possible, then bring it back to the center and across the body. Complete all the reps for one leg before facing the opposite direction and working the other leg.

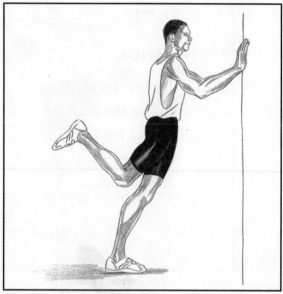

Trail Leg Windmill Stretch (1)

TRAIL LEG WINDMILL

Stand on your right leg and extend your arms in front of you touching a wall. Lift your right leg

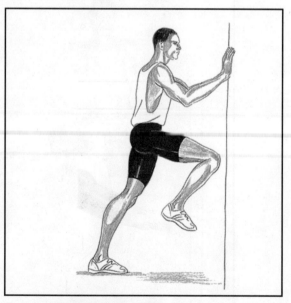

Trail Leg Windmill Stretch (2)

and move it back and forth, bending your knee as you do so. Perform all the reps with one leg before standing on your other leg to work the opposite leg.

LUNGE EXCHANGE

Also known as the "mountain climber," this stretch is more work than relaxation. Assume the start position shown, then quickly switch legs so that your left foot is in front. Perform fifteen to twenty reps, exchanging legs as you do so.

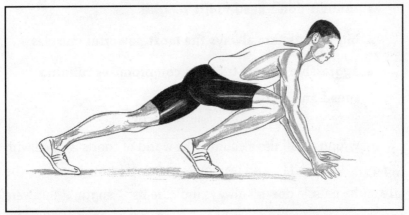

Lunge Exchange Stretch (1)

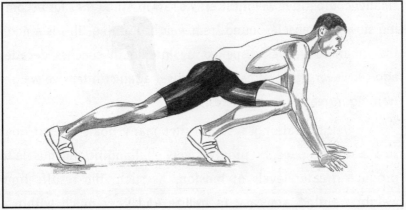

Lunge Exchange Stretch (2)

COMPONENT TWO
▲ STRENGTH TRAINING

Track and field athletes are a decidedly different group from, say, football players and weightlifters. As a general rule, most runners and jumpers are lean, and most throwers are big and muscular. Because of these obvious physical differences, many people make several assumptions about lifting weights. Among these are:

▲ **runners don't need to lift weights**

▲ **big muscles are always the most powerful muscles**

▲ **aggressive weight training compromises running speed and flexibility**

Wrong on all three counts. The world of sports is filled with big guys who run fast and lean guys with incredible strength. The size of the muscle doesn't always indicate its strength; if this were true, then bodybuilders would be stronger than the significantly smaller competitive weightlifters we saw in Atlanta. As for becoming slow and muscle-bound from weight training, this is a myth that, thankfully, was dispelled by intelligent coaches decades ago. However, there remains a mindset against intensive weight training in many track athletes.

Weight training accomplishes many goals, and it does so at a turtle's pace, by progressively challenging the muscle to produce greater levels of tension. As such, the results from weight training are easy to gauge and very much within a person's control. To be afraid to lift weights because you think in two weeks' time you'll look like a bodybuilder is ludicrous. Just ask the guys with the really big muscles and they'll tell you it can't happen overnight. There is of course the issue of steroids, which can produce dramatic changes. But this is a book about people serious about getting into the best shape of their lives. Steroids are not part of a *true* athlete's regimen because their effects are short-lived and counterproductive to living a long, vital, and athletic life.

There is overwhelming evidence from the sports of weightlifting and powerlifting that it is possible to significantly improve strength without increasing body weight. Fear of weight training will have a negative effect on your performance, yet it is doubtful that any type of athlete will suffer by gaining a few pounds of lean muscle mass.

Weight training can be performed in many different styles to accomplish different results. If you look at most athletes and their coaches, you'll usually see a similarity in body types. This is because the two are following similar training programs, which produce the same end results. In fact, I can usually tell what part of the country an athlete is from just by his or her general shape and build. For example, the Midwest tends to turn out bigger athletes because they put more emphasis on heavy weight training in their routines.

The strength-training portion of my conditioning program involves a three-day-per-week weight-training regimen in the gym. I generally like to use high repetitions, about twelve to fifteen, and about three sets, especially for the exercises that work the upper body. Depending upon your strength level and the exercise you're performing, you may need to perform fewer repetitions and more sets.

My weight-training regimen includes the Power Clean. The Power Clean develops strength and power. Because it requires a considerable amount of technique to master, it is best to have a qualified coach teach it to you. For that reason, I've eliminated it from my suggested routine here, but I have provided an extensive section on how it is performed. If you have a qualified coach or trainer, I strongly recommend that you learn this lift; and after you've learned it, include it in your routine.

Because your body adapts quickly to any specific weight training system, your weight training workouts need to be constantly monitored and modified. The monitoring lets you continue to make incremental gains; the modifications allow you to stay on a program to accomplish your goals.

The first question newcomers to weight training ask is, "How much should I lift?" This can't be answered until you begin a program, because you need to assess the amount of weight that challenges you in any given exercise. Start out light, then work your way up until you find weights that challenge your strength— the weights that you can lift for only one or two repetitions. Then you're ready to assess your proper loads. I generally like to use a weight that allows me to just barely complete the last three repetitions of my last set, but I don't resort to potentially harmful cheating techniques to use more weight or finish that final rep. I always strive to increase the weight slightly, but I keep the reps and sets constant.

DAN O'BRIEN'S WEIGHT WORKOUT

My weight-training program is a total body strength routine. I vary it according to what equipment is available at the facility where I'm training, and sometimes according to my mood. I also use an extensive arsenal of abdominal exercises. I once heard Muhammad Ali say that he did sit-ups until his abs hurt, then he started counting. I have the same philosophy, often doing a set of ab work in between each two major muscle groups, for a total of six to eight sets in one workout.

My routine is just that: mine. I keep the overall workout schedule consistent because I'm juggling so many training variables in a given week, and I don't want to be so fatigued from overworking one component of fitness that it adversely affects another. I heartily endorse the philosophy that it's better to be undertrained than overtrained. My point is that this is an ideal routine for a world champion gold medal decathlete in his early thirties who plans on reaching 9,000 points before he retires. In other words, it's ideal for me, but may not be ideal for anyone else. If you feel the need to make adjustments, do so.

Academic journals refer to weight training as *progressive resistance exercise.* By incrementally increasing the tension on a muscle, you cause it to adapt by growing and strengthening. For bodybuilders and weightlifters, this principle is employed to its fullest, with gains in strength or size occurring regularly, often noticeably with every other workout for beginners. These athletes have also discovered that muscles need to be shocked into growth—not by an outside electrical impulse, but by variety, as the body will adapt to any single workout protocol. Therefore, if you want to see major gains in size and strength from a weight-training routine on a continual basis, you'll need to incorporate both progressive increases into resistance and variety into your program.

I perform this program three times a week and never spend more than one hour in the gym.

This routine is an adjunct to my event training. There are many specific exercises and routines that you may choose to incorporate to improve a specific aspect of performance. This is a general conditioning routine that I use to enhance my track and field performance. You can use it as a starting point or even as a maintenance routine.

Dan's Ultimate Weight-Training Routine

	Sets	Reps
Alternate Dumbbell Curl	3	10-12
Dumbbell Isolation Curl	3	10-12
Flat Bench Dumbbell Press	3	10-12
Dumbbell Fly	3	10-12
Behind the Neck Press	3	10-12
Upright Rows	3	10-12

Dan's Ultimate Weight-Training Routine (continued)

	Sets	Reps	
Lat Pulldowns	3	10-12	(not shown)
Seated Cable Row	3	10-12	(not shown)
Deep Squat	3	10-12	
Forward Lunge	3	10-12	
Hamstring Curl	4	15-20	(not shown)

Calves are stretched with calf raises during warm-up drills before track training. Abdominals are worked in between major muscle group sets, using the following variety of exercises performed to failure:

Feet-up crunch

Oblique crunch

Legs crossed crunch

Bicycle

Knee-ups off bench

Low back stretch

▲ Weight Training Exercises

Alternate Dumbbell Curl

Although I perform several types of curls in my workout, I especially like performing curls in an alternating fashion because it is more biomechancially specific to the arm action used in running. This exercise is a basic bicep builder.

From a standing position, grasp a pair of dumbbells and turn your wrists so that your palms are facing away from you. Look straight ahead and maintain good posture with your chest up and shoulders back. Curl one of the dumbbells until the plates touch your shoulders, and as you lower it, begin curling the other dumbbell. Do not swing the dumbbells, and only lower your arms until they are straight—do not hyperextend at the elbow.

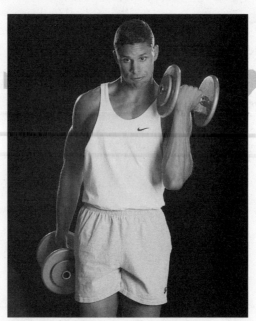

Alternate Dumbbell Curl Excercise

DAN'S TIPS: Although you can lift more weight by swinging the weights and leaning backward during this exercise, don't! That technique is not only stressful on the lower back, but also alters the biomechanics of the movement so that the muscles are not trained properly.

BEHIND-THE-NECK PRESS

This exercise works the shoulders. Perform it by sitting on the edge of a bench with your feet slightly more than shoulder width

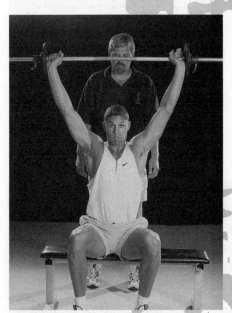

apart. Place a barbell behind your head on your shoulders, not on the neck region (either by removing the barbell from supports or by having a partner hand it to you), and position your grip slightly wider than shoulder width apart. Point the elbows down.

Begin the movement by pressing the weight overhead to arm's length

Behind-The-Neck Press Excercise

and then slowly lowering it again to your shoulders. Look straight ahead while pressing and keep your chin slightly retracted (tucked in) throughout the movement, avoiding the tendency to poke your head forward and down.

DAN'S TIPS: Although the bulk of a weight training program for an athlete should be with free weights, I prefer performing this exercise with a Smith machine, which consists of a barbell that rides up and down on a rail.

DEEP SQUAT

It's often been said in the weight room that if you don't have the squat in your program, you don't have a program. The squat is the single best exercise for the major muscle groups of the lower body. Although there has been some controversy in the past over whether the squat may be harmful to the knees, credible research has shown that regular squatting is in fact one of the best ways to *prevent* knee injuries.

Resistance for the squat is provided by resting a barbell across the back of your shoulders. Because you can squat with more weight than you can lift from the floor, you will need to begin

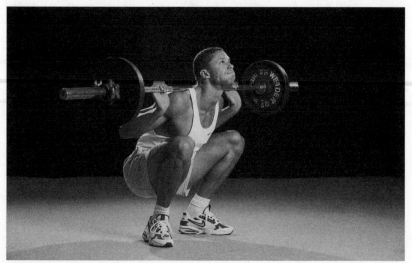

Deep Squat Excercise (1)

the exercise by removing the barbell from a set of supports, such as those provided in a power rack.

Assume the start position by spreading your feet shoulder width apart, arching your back slightly, and looking straight ahead and slightly upward. Begin by taking a deep breath and then slowly bend your knees, forcing them outward and in line with your feet. Lower your hips until your thighs are below parallel to the floor, and then return to the start, looking slightly up as you do. Although there is no problem going all the way to the bottom as I do, you should never bounce out of the bottom position or round your back.

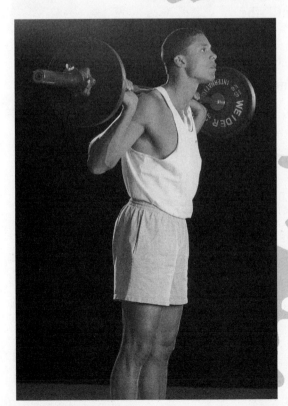

Deep Squat Excercise (2)

DAN'S TIPS: If you cannot keep your heels on the floor (or if you have to lean excessively forward as you descend), you need to stretch your calves and hip flexors or try a slightly wider stance. In the meantime, you can compensate for this muscle tightness by elevating your heels with a small board.

DUMBBELL CURL

This is another exercise for the upper arms. From a standing position, grasp a pair of dumbbells and turn your wrists so that your palms are facing away from you. Look straight ahead and maintain good posture with your chest up and shoulders back. Curl both dumbbells until the plates touch your shoulders, then return to the start. Do not swing the dumbbells, and only lower your arms until they are straight—do not hyperextend at the elbow.

DAN'S TIPS: Using a weight belt while you perform this exercise encourages you to maintain an upright posture and not swing the weights.

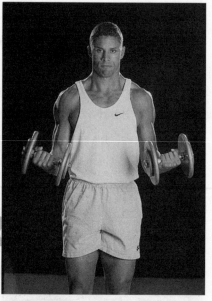

Dumbbell Curl Excercise (1)

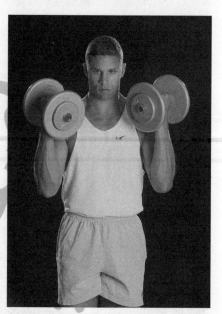

Dumbbell Curl Excercise (2)

DUMBBELL FLY

Because I use this exercise primarily as a stretch for the chest area, I don't use heavy weights. Hold two light dumbbells and sit down on a flat bench, resting one end of each plate on your thighs. Kick the weights up to your shoulders with your legs, one at a time, and then lie back on the bench. Press the dumbbells to arm's length with the palms facing each

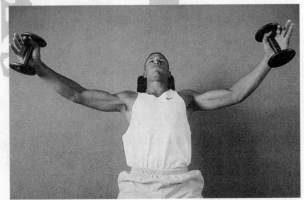

Dumbbell Fly Excercise (1)

other. Keeping the elbows slightly bent, lower the dumbbells out to the side in an arc until your upper arms are parallel to the floor. Slowly moving the dumbbells in an arc, without jerking, return to the start position.

DAN'S TIPS: Although you will see many individuals allow the dumbbells to drop below parallel in the bottom

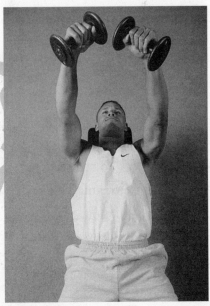

Dumbbell Fly Excercise (2)

position, don't copy their technique. The shoulder is especially susceptible to injury when you do this.

DUMBBELL ROW

This is a great exercise for strengthening the back. Grasp a dumbbell in your right hand. Place your left knee on a flat bench, your left foot on the floor, and your left arm on the bench. Bend forward from the waist so that your back is parallel to the floor. Holding the dumbbell with your palm down, perform the exercise by pulling the dumbbell to the middle portion of your chest in one smooth motion. Repeat for the other side.

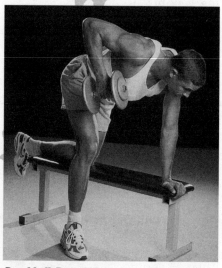

Dumbbell Row (1)

DAN'S TIPS: To reinforce your grip, you should use straps when you start using heavy weights for this exercise.

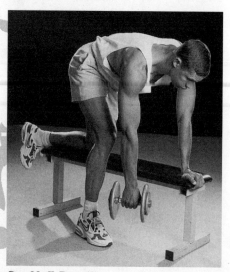

Dumbbell Row (2)

DUMBBELL ISOLATION CURL

This is another biceps exercise. I often interchange biceps exercises to keep my routine interesting, but will at times perform all of these variations in a single routine. Grasp a dumbbell, sit down on the end of a flat bench, and spread your feet slightly apart. Rest your right elbow against the inside of your right thigh and place your left hand on your left knee for balance. Without lifting your arm from your thigh, curl the weight upward until the plates touch your shoulders, then lower the weight to the start. Repeat for the other side.

DAN'S TIPS: At the top position, try to turn the wrists inward slightly to increase the contraction of the biceps.

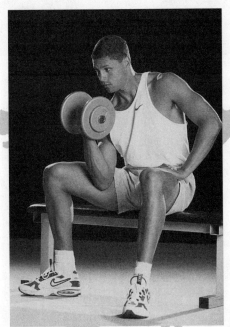

Dumbbell Isolation Curl

FLAT BENCH DUMBBELL PRESS

In addition to developing arm and shoulder power for the shot put, the flat bench dumbbell press helps your arm action in running by working the triceps—especially the long head—and the front part of the shoulders (anterior deltoids).

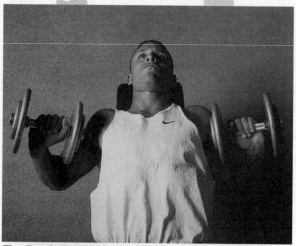

Flat Bench Dumbbell Press (1)

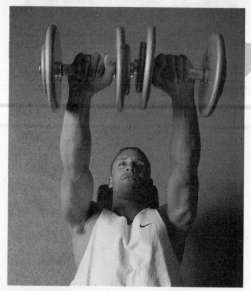

Flat Bench Dumbbell Press (2)

Grasp two dumbbells and sit down on a flat bench, resting one end of each plate on your thighs. Kick the weights up to your shoulders with your legs, one dumbbell at a time, and then lie back on the bench. Twist your hands so that your palms face your feet, and flare your elbows slightly out to the sides and down.

From this starting position, press the weights upward in a slight arc so that they come together at the top. Pause in this fully contracted position and then slowly return the weights to your shoulders. At first this may feel awkward because many of the smaller muscles of the shoulders have to work especially hard to stabilize the dumbbells, but the proper technique should come naturally after your second or third workout.

DAN'S TIPS: When you use heavy weights with this exercise it becomes difficult to lift them to the start position yourself. If this is the case, lie back on the bench and have a spotter hand you the weights.

FORWARD LUNGE

The Forward Lunge works your legs throughout a full range of motion and in a manner that is biomechanically specific to running. As such, it is one of the best exercises for increasing your stride length and leg thrust, as well as decreasing your risk of injury.

Place a barbell behind your head, resting it on the shoulders. Hold the bar with your hands shoulder width apart, elbows pointed down. Begin by taking a large step forward, keeping

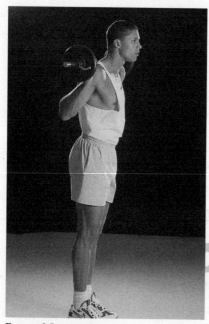

Forward Lunge (1)

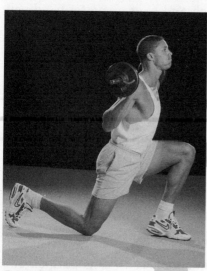

Forward Lunge (2)

your head and chest up and looking straight ahead or slightly up. Now bend your knees and lower your hips until your back knee drops to a point just above the floor—never let your knee touch the floor. When I perform this exercise, I lower my trailing knee to the floor; as a highly trained athlete I keep my concentration focused on the movement and stay in complete control. I don't recommend this technique for other people.

Complete the exercise by pushing off with your forward leg and then stepping back when the knee is completely straight. Repeat for the opposite leg. A single repetition for the lunge consists of one complete movement for each leg.

As this exercise becomes more natural, you will be able to descend directly into the lowest position in one smooth motion.

DAN'S TIPS: Because your back is held vertically during this exercise, you should not feel any significant pressure on your lower back. If you do, you're probably leaning forward during the exercise. Also, if you still feel unstable after performing it for several sessions, try turning your front foot out five to ten degrees.

HAMSTRING CURL

Hamstring work is absolutely essential to a track-and-field athlete's weight training routine, and not just because it prevents injury to this major leg muscle. Being able to bend the knee quickly and contract it strongly during the follow-through of the running motion enables you to move the entire leg faster, resulting in an increase in stride frequency.

Performing the hamstring curl re-quires access to a leg curl machine, which comes in three major varieties: seated, standing, and prone. The seated and standing varieties have become the most popular, as with the prone variety there is a tendency to arch your back as you perform the exercise, creating a stress that may aggravate back pain. The basic technique points for using these machines, however, are the same.

Regardless of the type of machine you have access to, position yourself so that your knees are in line with the center of the pulley apparatus and your ankles rest behind the pads. On the prone leg curl machine, your knees should extend at least an inch beyond the bench (to avoid compressing your kneecaps). On the seated leg curl machine, your knees should be in line with the

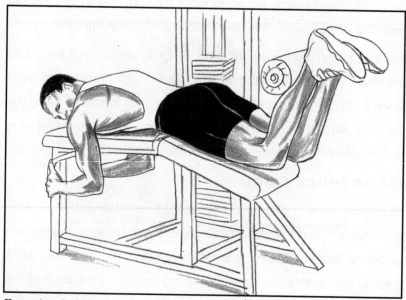

Hamstring Curl (1)

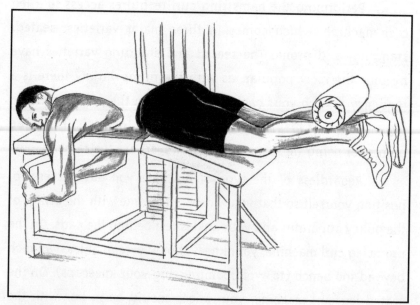

Hamstring Curl (2)

pulley apparatus. Also, always keep your toes pointed so your calves don't cramp.

Begin the exercise by slowly pulling your ankles toward your buttocks; ideally, the pad should touch your buttocks. Hold the peak contraction briefly before returning to the start position. Avoid the tendency to arch your lower back or jerk the weight at the start of the exercise in an attempt to lift more weight.

DAN'S TIPS: It's important to achieve a full range of motion on this exercise. If you find that you cannot do so, your hip flexors may be tight, the weight you are using may be too heavy, or the machine you are using may be poorly designed.

LAT PULLDOWN

This back-building exercise requires the use of a lat pulldown machine or a high pulley with a flat bench. Grasp the bar with a shoulder-width grip, and then sit on the machine so that your shoulders are positioned directly underneath the cable. This is an important point, as sitting too far away from the machine will cause you to poke your head forward as you pull the weight down, and also cause you to flex your wrists, which can strain the forearm muscles and put excessive stress on the elbows. Begin by pulling the bar to your collarbone and leaning slightly back until the bar touches your collarbone. Pause in this fully contracted position and then slowly return to the start.

DAN'S TIPS: This should be a natural movement; do not use the technique advocated by many exercise specialists in which you fully retract your shoulders and then follow through with the

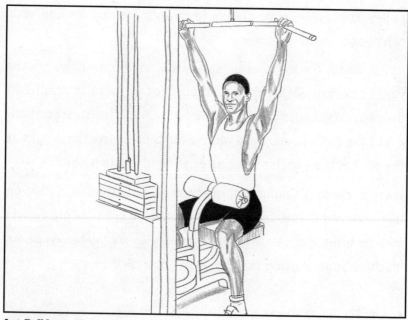

Lat Pulldown (1)

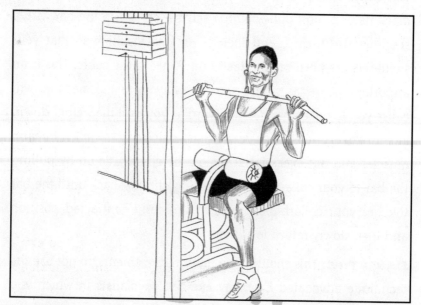

Lat Pulldown (2)

arms—this is especially stressful to the upper back muscles and may eventually cause injury.

SEATED CABLE ROW

This exercise for strengthening the back muscles requires the use of a low row machine or a low pulley cable apparatus. Sit down and bend your knees slightly—do not lock them, as this can overstress your lower back. Keep your back slightly arched and tuck in your chin slightly. Begin by leaning forward slightly from the hips, then pull the shoulders back while bending the arms. Your arms should be positioned a few inches away from your sides as you do this. Keep pulling, leaning backward and allowing the bar to touch the middle of your chest. At this point, finish the movement by squeezing the shoulder blades together. As you perform this entire movement, keep your head in line with your torso—do not poke your head forward.

DAN'S TIPS: I like to put my feet behind me because I feel it better isolates the back muscles.

TRICEPS PULLOVER

This is a fantastic exercise for the shoulder, upper back, and arm muscles that are used to throw the javelin. I especially like it because it puts the upper back and shoulder muscles through such a long range of motion.

Lie face up on a flat bench and press a barbell to arm's length (or remove it from the bench supports). Using a shoulder-width grip and keeping your upper arm stationary, lower the weight until it's level with your forehead, then continue the

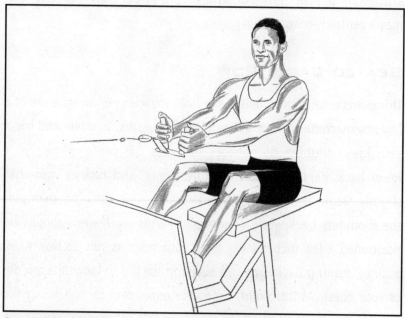

Seated Cable Row (1)

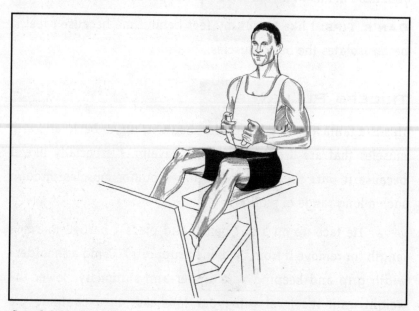

Seated Cable Row (2)

downward motion by allowing the upper arm to drop to the position shown. Reverse the procedure to return to the start.

DAN'S TIPS: To avoid neck strain, your head should be fully supported by the bench, not allowed to hang over the edge. Also, if this exercise bothers your wrists, try performing it with an "E-Z curl" barbell, which is a barbell that has a jigsaw shape in the center.

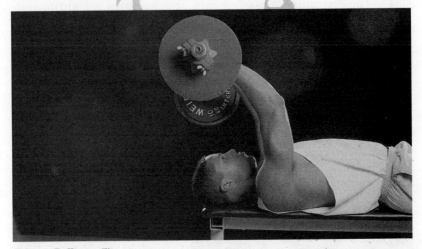

Triceps Pullover (1)

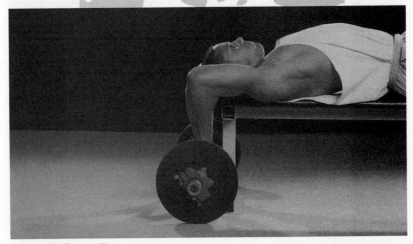

Triceps Pullover (2)

Upright Row

The upper body muscles, especially the trapezius, contribute up to fifteen percent of your power in jumping. The upright row is an excellent exercise to develop these muscles.

Grasp a barbell with a close grip, palms facing your body, and curl your wrists so that your elbows flare out to the sides. Look straight ahead. Begin the exercise by shrugging your shoulders and bending your arms until the barbell touches your collarbone. Your elbows should be coming up, not back. Now reverse the movement, returning the bar to arm's length and then lowering it to the floor.

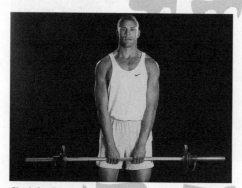

Upright Row (1)

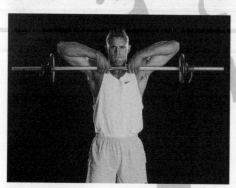

Upright Row (2)

DAN'S TIPS: If you're not able to bring the weight to your collarbone, it could be due to a lack of flexibility, but it probably means that you're using too much weight. Also, if you have a difficult time holding on to the bar during the last few reps, use lifting straps to reinforce your grip.

▲ ABDOMINAL AND LOWER BACK EXERCISES

BACK EXTENSION

For the high jump, it's especially important to work the lower back muscles through a full range of motion in order to get into the proper position over the bar. The back extension fulfills this requirement, and is generally considered a very safe exercise.

Lie face down with your arms against your sides, palms up. Begin by squeezing your buttocks, lifting your head, arms, shoulders and lower legs off the floor as shown. At the top position you need to concentrate on squeezing your shoulder blades together. Lower to the start and repeat.

DAN'S TIPS: If you have a forward head posture in which your chin pokes forward and you have an excessive hump in the upper back, you should make two small modifications to the

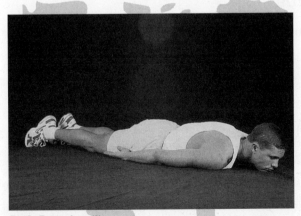

Back Extension (1)

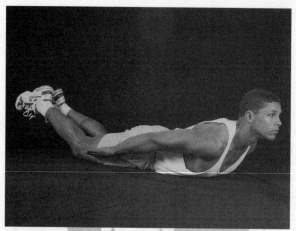

Back Extension (2)

exercise. First, instead of keeping your palms up throughout the movement, externally rotate your hands (twist them outward so that your palms point up) as you lift your chest off the floor. Also, look down as you perform the movement, keeping your chin retracted (tucked in).

BICYCLE

Strong hip flexors are a must for a sprinter or high jumper because these muscles lift the knee up. The bicycle is a great exercise because the legs are worked alternately, just as they function in these activities.

Flex your hips and knees to ninety degrees. Place your hands by your sides. Begin the exercise by extending the left knee while simultaneously driving the right knee in the opposite direction toward the shoulders. Continue alternating in this manner until all reps have been completed.

DAN'S TIPS: As you get comfortable with the technique of this exercise, you can increase the difficulty by using ankle weights.

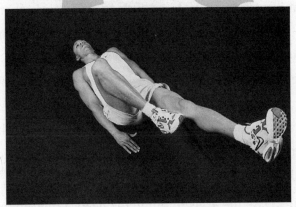

Bicycle

FEET-UP CRUNCH

This exercise isolates the upper abdominals far better than the conventional sit-up, which primarily works the hip flexor muscles that lift the legs. To even more effectively isolate the upper abdominals, drape your lower legs over the top of a bench so your upper legs are perpendicular to the floor.

Beginners should perform the crunch with their arms at their sides; intermediates can place

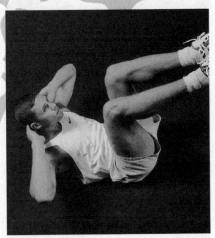

Feet-Up Crunch

their hands across their chests; and those who are advanced can place their hands on the sides of their heads, just behind the ears. Perform the crunch by tightening your lower abdominal muscles and curling your torso just to the point where your shoulders leave the floor. Do not tuck your chin against your chest; instead, leave a few inches between your jaw and collarbone. When you return to the start, let your shoulders and head make full contact with the mat before performing another repetition. This ensures that the muscles are worked through a full range of motion and minimizes the stress on your neck and upper back.

DAN'S TIPS: Use the arms to guide the head, rather than trying to make the exercise easier by pulling on the head.

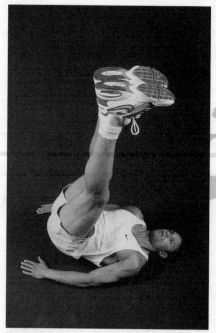

Hip Lift

HIP LIFT

This exercise will work the important muscles of the lower abdominal region which help you maintain an upright running position. Also, by helping to balance out the pull of the powerful hip flexor muscles, the hip lift prevents the excessive back arch you see in many athletes that can contribute to back pain.

Lie on your back with your hands beside your hips and your legs perpendicular to the floor. Perform the exercise by lifting your hips upward as shown, minimizing the amount of leg swing, and return to the start.

DAN'S TIPS: You can increase the difficulty of this exercise with ankle weights, or by performing it on an incline.

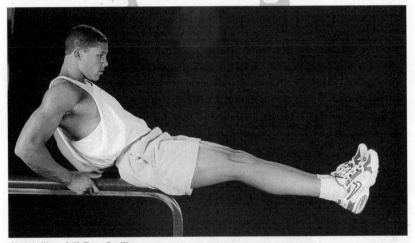

Knees-Ups Off Bench (1)

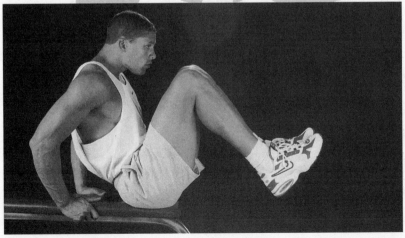

Knees-Ups Off Bench (2)

Knee-Ups Off Bench

This exercise is performed off the end of a stable bench. Position your hips at the end of a bench, holding on to the sides of the bench for stability. With your feet together, pull your knees to your chest and then extend them out to the start position. Do not arch your back as you perform this movement; instead, keep it relatively straight or slightly rounded.

Dan's Tips: You can increase the difficulty of this exercise by holding a dumbbell between your feet.

Legs-crossed Crunch

This version of the crunch more effectively isolates the upper abdominals because it prevents the hip flexors from contributing to the movement. Cross your legs and place your hands on the

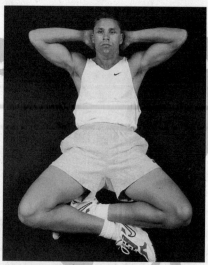

Legs-Crossed Crunch

sides of your head, just behind the ears. Perform the crunch by tightening your lower abdominal muscles and curling your torso to the point where your shoulders leave the floor. Do not tuck your chin against your chest as you crunch; instead, leave a few inches between your jaw and collarbone. When you return to the start, let your shoulders and head make full contact with the floor before performing another repetition.

DAN'S TIPS: Because of the position of the legs, there is a strong tendency to arch your back while performing this exercise. To counter this action, which places unnatural stress on the spine, concentrate on flattening your back as you come up.

OBLIQUE CRUNCH

Strong obliques, the muscles on the sides of your waist, provide power in throwing the javelin and shot put, and help maintain stability when you run. The oblique crunch is an excellent exercise to isolate these muscles.

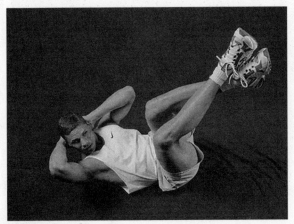

Oblique Crunch

This abdominal exercise begins just like the advanced version of the feet-up crunch, with your hands on the sides of your head, behind the ears. The difference is that as you start to come forward, you twist your head, neck and shoulders as a unit to bring your left elbow to your right knee. Slowly return to the starting position, and then reverse the movement for the abdominal muscles on the other side of the trunk.

DAN'S TIPS: The exercise is considered complete when you fully contract the obliques. However, some individuals may not be able to touch their elbows to their knees because of anatomical limitations. Don't worry about it as long as you are able to feel a good contraction.

THE POWER CLEAN

The power clean can play an important part in a decathlete's conditioning. In addition to working the major muscle groups involved in running and jumping, this dynamic exercise emphasizes the development of fast twitch muscle fibers. It also teaches the muscles to work in synergy, unlike many isolation exercises that require little coordination.

The power clean is a multi-joint exercise that requires good coaching to achieve perfect technique, and I strongly recommend that you seek help from a qualified strength coach if you've never performed it. Nevertheless, the fact is that the power clean can be learned rather quickly by anyone. The best way to learn it is to break the lift down into its component parts and, after each part is mastered, combine them to complete the lift.

The most difficult segment of the power clean is to master the lift from the floor to the mid-thigh. As such, it's better to teach the lift "from the top down," working on the simpler components before addressing the more complex ones. Even if the lift is never mastered from the floor, considerable benefit can be attained by performing only the second portion of the lift. Also, to speed up the learning process, it can help to practice the lift in front of a mirror.

The first step in learning the power clean is to grip the barbell with a hand-spacing slightly wider than shoulder width. Stand up, rest the barbell on your mid-thighs, and look straight ahead. Now lift your chest up so there's a slight arch in your

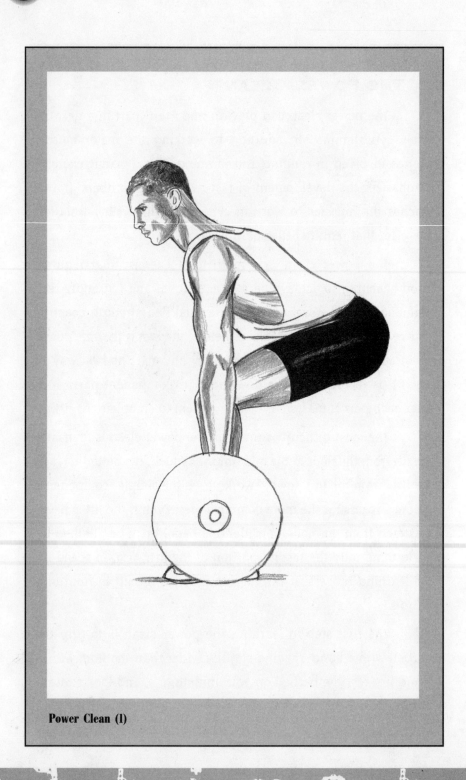

Power Clean (1)

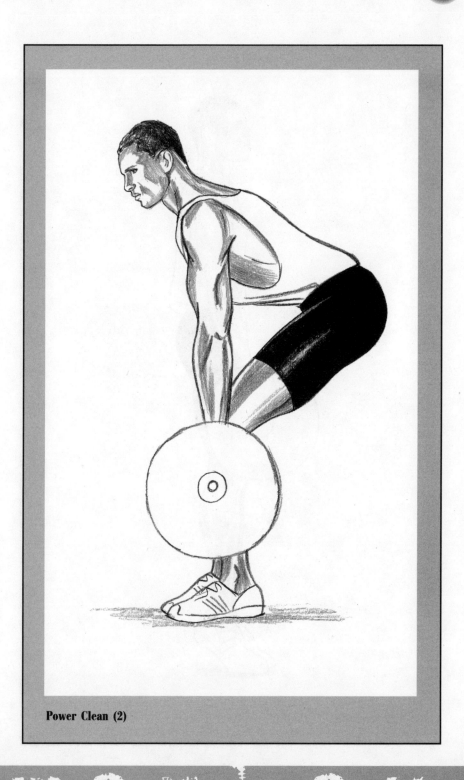

Power Clean (2)

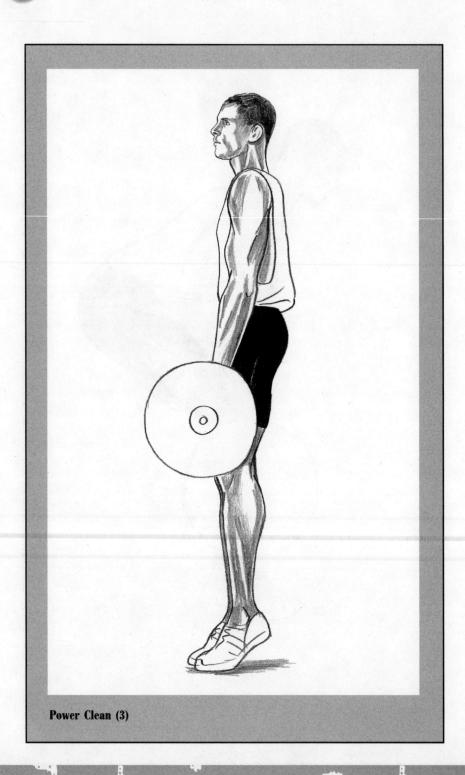

Power Clean (3)

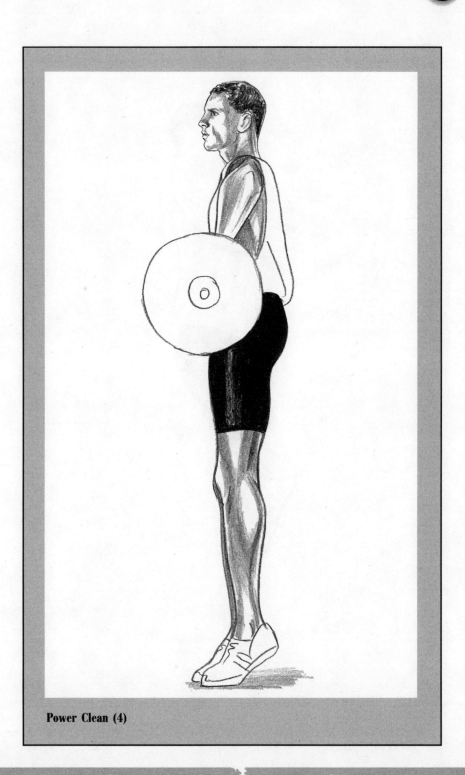

Power Clean (4)

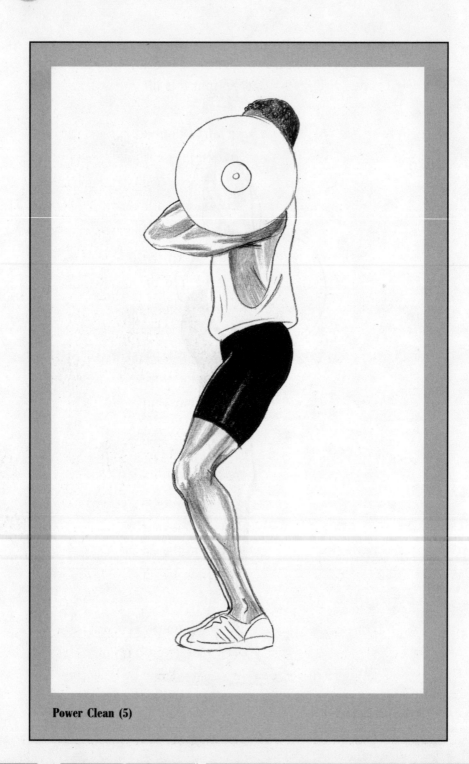

Power Clean (5)

lower back, pull your shoulders back, and curl your wrists so that your elbows flare out to the side. From this fully-erect position, lean forward slightly so that your shoulders extend slightly in front of the bar, and position the barbell on your thighs so that you feel the majority of your body weight on the middle of your foot. This is what is known as the *power position*, and is the point where you begin the maximum acceleration of the barbell. Spend at least ten minutes getting comfortable with this position.

The next step is to learn how to lift the weight from the power position to the shoulders. Move into the power position, then straighten your legs and follow through by shrugging your shoulders, ending your arms so that the bar touches the bottom of your ribcage. Lower the bar to the power position and repeat several times until you feel comfortable with this motion. Again, the basic concept is to straighten your legs and follow through by shrugging your shoulders.

The next step is to continue the upright row by turning your wrists over at the top and catching the weight on the top of your shoulders. At the catch position it's important to thrust your shoulders forward so that the weight rests on the muscles, and to keep your hands relaxed. Lower the weight to the power position and continue working on making this motion feel natural, each time trying to increase your speed.

The last step in learning the lift from the power position involves explosively using the major muscle grounds of the back, hips, and legs to thrust the weight upward. From a fully erect position, lower the bar to the power position and then "kick" the weight upward with a powerful extension. What you'll find is that this *counter motion* creates a recoil effect that will dramatically increase the acceleration of the bar.

At this point, I recommend devoting several training sessions to just working on lifting from the power position. When you feel comfortable enough, and are performing the lift with considerable speed, then you can proceed to lifting the weight from the floor.

The first step in learning how to master the power clean from the floor is to stand facing the bar, placing your toes a few inches under and in front of the bar (slightly less if you're tall). Now arch your back, bend your knees, and grasp the bar. Move your head in line with your back so that your focus is on a spot on the floor about six feet ahead of you. To place your hips in proper alignment, move your knees so they are in line with your elbows, with the bar slightly touching your shins (or, if you're tall, about an inch away). This will position your lower body to maximize use of the lower body muscles.

The next step is to bring the barbell from the start position to the power position. Begin by holding your breath and then straightening just your legs so that the bar is brought to the power position. As this occurs you'll see that to keep the weight close to your body, the bar needs to travel slightly backwards. Also, as the knees straighten, you cannot allow your back to extend significantly. Repeat this dead lift technique several times. The major technique point is not to pull up the weight so fast that you round your back—only pull as fast as good technique will allow.

When you feel comfortable with the power clean dead lift from the floor, the final step is to combine the two portions of the lift. Thus, you would perform the dead lift and, when you reach the power position, kick the weight to the shoulders. Do this slowly at first, gradually increasing the second portion of the lift. As you perfect the movement, you will get less of a bump off the thighs and more of a brush when you hit the power position. You will also be able to perform the lift faster.

As far as repetitions, most athletes use fewer repetitions with heavy weight. Performing more reps requires that you have exceptional technique and concentration; however, if you choose to perform the lift from just the power position, the significantly shorter range of motion will allow you to perform more reps comfortably.

COMPONENT THREE
▲ BALLISTIC STRENGTH TRAINING

Resistance training with weights will improve your physique, increase your overall muscular strength and, to some extent, enhance your ability to perform endurance activities. In sports where running is key to success, the lower body strength developed from weight training will increase the amount of force your legs can apply to the ground. In the early stages of athletic development, this strength translates into better sprinting and jumping ability.

Upper body strength is also important for running and jumping to help you control the torque generated in your legs, which is why top sprinters emphasize upper body work in their weight workouts and have the physiques to prove it. (In fact, at a body weight of 173 pounds, Ben Johnson could bench-press 420 pounds and run the 100 meters in 9.79, which is .05 seconds faster than the officially recognized world record. Although Johnson used steroids, being able to run that fast does prove that upper body strength may play an even more important role in sprinting than was previously thought.)

Weight training is important to all track athletes, but running and jumping at my level of competition requires emphasis on a more *specific* type of strength that can't be accomplished with traditional weight training. It's what I call *ballistic strength*.

Although exercise scientists often use the term "speed-strength" with its numerous subcomponents such as reactive ability and explosive strength, I prefer the simple term "ballistic

strength" because it effectively expresses the concept of dynamic, rapid movement. Think of ballistic strength as that athletic
quality that rockets you out of the starting block or springs you
off the floor to dunk a basketball. Ballistic strength is that extra
edge that separates the competitor from the participant, and the
champion from the competitor.

Developing ballistic strength requires you to perform special exercises and drills that cause the muscles to produce as much
force as possible, as quickly as possible. The drawback to most
weight-training exercises is that they have to be performed slowly, especially in single-joint exercises that isolate the muscles.
Also, in multi-joint exercises, such as squats, much of the exercise
must be spent decelerating the weight to ease safely into the end
position. In contrast, most sports require the muscles to contract
powerfully throughout their entire length, to follow through with
the motion. Now don't get me wrong—weight training is essential,
but for peak athletic performance you also need to concentrate on
training what are known as *fast-twitch muscle fibers.*

Fast-twitch muscle fibers are capable of rapid, intense
contractions and are the primary types of fibers used in running
for speed, jumping and throwing. In contrast, *slow-twitch muscle
fibers* don't contract as hard, but can contract at a consistent level
for extended periods. An individual's fast- and slow-twitch muscle ratio is largely determined at birth—mine definitely favors
fast-twitch, which is one reason that sprinting is easy for me, and
accounts for the fact that I will never be a good marathon runner.
(Likewise, Florence Griffith tried marathon running after breaking
world records in the 100 and 200 meters in the 1988 Olympics, but

has not come close to world-class standards.) Regardless of the ratio of muscle fibers you were born with, through long-term training you can enhance the performance of either. The key here is *long-term*. I see athletes in other sports work on ballistic strength two months out of the year and then expect that training to carry through to the next year. It doesn't. That is why track athletes must train year-round on conditioning and should embrace the concept of goal setting.

To enhance the performance of the fast-twitch fibers responsible for ballistic strength, I perform numerous speed-specific training drills. They are based on a continuum of activities that range from low intensity activities like skipping (which I now only use to warm up) to more intense activities like box jumps.

The most advanced form of ballistic training is *plyometrics*, developed by Russian scientist Yuri Verkhoshansky more than thirty years ago. Plyometrics involve extremely dynamic movements that provide a mechanical shock stimulation, which forces a muscle to produce as much tension as rapidly as possible. An example of a plyometric training exercise is dropping off a sixteen-inch-high box while keeping the legs relatively relaxed, and then jumping as high as possible immediately after you land. For the upper body, a push-up in which you clap between repetitions and rebound immediately is an example of a plyometric training exercise. However, these specific plyometric exercises are considered highly advanced, and some athletes may never reach the level where they will be ready for this type of intense training. Those that do try them before they are ready often get disappointing results and risk injury. It's important for athletes to communicate with their coaches, constantly reevaluate their physical preparation, and plan their workouts carefully.

BOUNDING DRILLS

One of the best exercises to improve ballistic strength is bounding. Bounding exercises are running drills that emphasize specific components of running, such as hip extension or knee lift. They use exaggerated forms of running and allow you to work on all the nuances of sprinting and hurdling. Bounding is absolutely essential to sprinting.

Bounding drills, combined with fast feet drills, are designed to increase the speed of muscular contraction—the so-called stride frequency. This is the factor that separates great sprinters from good sprinters. The improvement of a sprinter involves the refinement and strengthening of the natural running movement. The object of these drills is to get rid of wasteful movements while making efficient movements stronger and smoother. Therefore, when you perform these drills, the motions should feel natural and relaxed—not tense as when lifting weights.

Good arm action is essential in bounding. During sprinting drills the hands should be by the pockets, brushing slightly, elbows bent. The shoulders should be down and relaxed, rolling backward and forward with the pumping of the arms, and the torso and head are held high—the "running tall" posture. During the jumps you need to bring your arms up as your body comes up, then recover and be in position for the next jump. During alternate leg hops you need to pay special attention to the dorsi-flexion of the foot. Always focus on the next step, skip, jump, or hurdle—for every step taken, apply equal attention to making certain the landing is in total preparation of the next step.

At the end of my lower-body days (twice a week), I finish up with several field drills. I'll do hurdle hops beginning with double-leg hops, then single, then alternate. I like to use hurdles of different heights in order to keep my mind involved in the hops, constantly sizing up, gauging and working on precise performance. I usually finish off this workout with one-legged hops up stairs. Although earlier in my training I worked in the gym with plyometrics, I now find the high- and long-jump workouts are enough.

Both bounding and field drills increase an athlete's skill and effective coordination of the techniques involved in efficient performance of an activity. By increasing such mastery, an athlete's self-control is also enhanced. These drills require concentration, determination, pace judgment, and resistance to pain and fatigue.

Nothing replaces actual competition to learn how to control nervousness. Until you've been there, there is no way to recreate the actual tension and anxiety. When I no-heighted the pole vault in 1992, the fact that I hadn't been in actual competition for nearly a year prior played a big role. It caught me off balance; I lost my focus. I had never no-heighted before, and I've never since. I'll never know exactly what happened that day, but I have spent every day since then making certain it doesn't happen again.

▲ DAN'S TRACK AND FIELD DRILLS

ALTERNATE-LEG HOPS

These can also be done as alternate-leg hurdle hops.

Perform the exercise by hopping forward on one leg and then the other, swinging your arms alternately as you do. To perform with hurdles, place a series of low hurdles in a row, the height and distance between the hurdles based on your jumping ability. Stand in front of the first barrier.

DAN'S TIPS: When you first perform this exercise with hurdles, use the lowest possible hurdles you can find, only increasing the height when you feel comfortable with your technique.

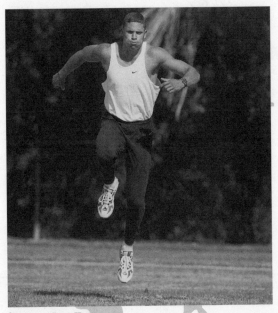

Alternate-Leg Hops

Box Jumps

These are performed in the gym and require a sturdy box that has a surface area of at least twenty-four inches. Stand in front of the box with your feet hip width apart or slightly wider and hands clasped behind your head. Bend your knees about ten degrees as you cock your arms backward, and then immediately jump onto the box.

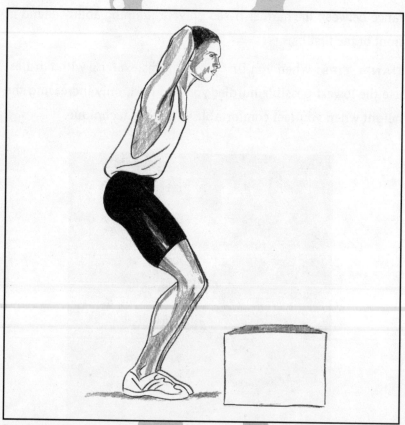

Box Jumps (1)

Make your landing as soft as possible. Step (don't jump) off the box and repeat for the recommended number of repetitions.

DAN'S TIPS: Make your landing as soft as possible, trying not to make any noise when you land, to minimize the stress on the knees.

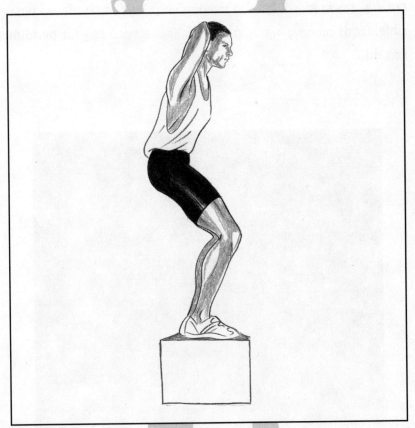

Box Jumps (2)

BUTT KICKS

This drill emphasizes a powerful contraction of the hamstrings and ideal alignment of the back leg in the recovery phase. For this drill, you keep your upper legs perpendicular to the ground and snap your lower legs back and up, kicking yourself in the rear with your heels. All the movement of the leg is from below the knee. Use an alternate arm swing.

DAN'S TIPS: In addition to moving your legs as rapidly as possible, focus on keeping your quadriceps relaxed as your perform this drill.

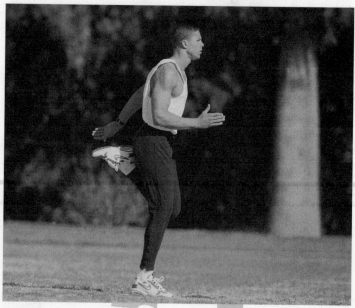

Butt Kicks

DOUBLE-LEG BOUNDS

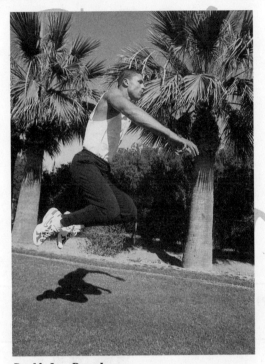

Double-Leg Bounds

This is a great exercise for overall leg, back and gluteal power and, when performed for longer distances, muscular endurance.

Stand with your feet shoulder width apart. Bend your knees, pull your arms back, and jump forward. As you jump, bring both arms forward and in front of you, and then pull them back as you prepare to land and jump again.

DAN'S TIPS: Just before you land, hold your breath and anticipate hitting the ground; exhale as you jump.

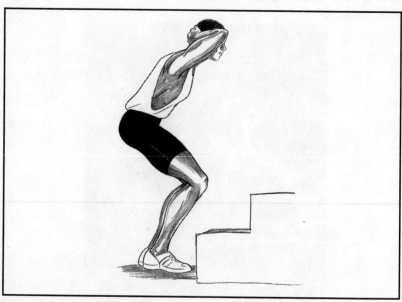

Double-Leg Hops Up Stairs (1)

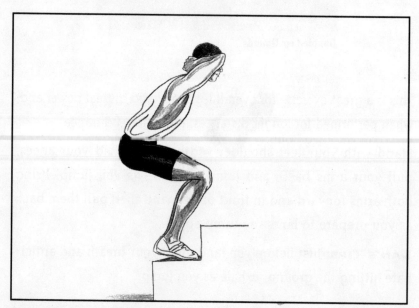

Double-Leg Hops Up Stairs (2)

DOUBLE-LEG HOPS UP STAIRS

These require a series of stairs such as you would find in a stadium or basketball gym. Stand at the bottom of the stairs. Hop up the stairs on both legs, with your hands clasped behind your head.

DAN'S TIPS: Always keep your eyes on the steps as you land, as it's easy to miss a step and fall when performing this exercise.

DOUBLE-LEG HURDLE HOPS

Place a series of low hurdles in a row, the height and distance apart of each hurdle based on your jumping ability. Stand in front

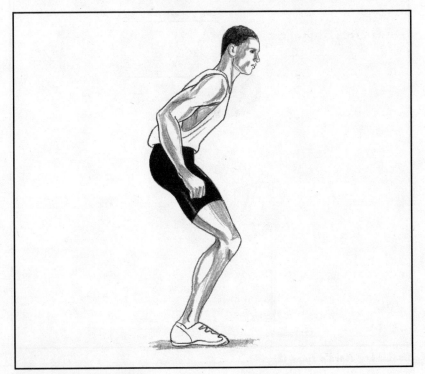

Double-Leg Hurdle Hops (1)

of the first barrier. Perform the exercise by hopping forward over the hurdles on both legs, swinging your arms back and forth as you do.

DAN'S TIPS: When you first perform this exercise with hurdles, use the lowest possible hurdles you can find, only increasing the height when you feel comfortable with your technique.

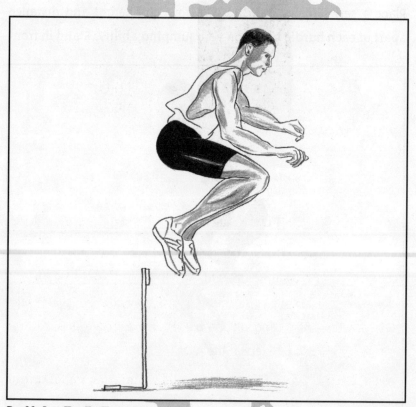

Double-Leg Hurdle Hops (2)

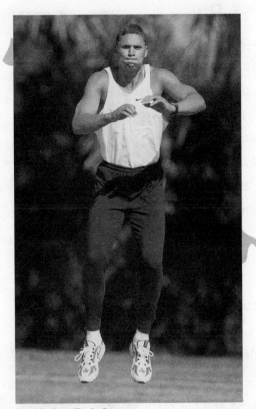

Double-Leg Tuck Jumps

DOUBLE-LEG TUCK JUMPS

Stand with your feet shoulder width apart. Bend your knees, pull your arms back, and jump upward, bringing both arms forward and pulling your knees to your chest. At the top position grasp your knees momentarily. Land on the balls of your feet, knees slightly bent, and immediately repeat the jump.

DAN'S TIPS: Just as in running and jumping, it's important to maintain an upright posture as you perform this exercise.

FAST FEET DRILL

This drill increases stride frequency by forcing you to get your feet off the ground quickly by powerfully contracting your hip flexors. It is performed by lifting your feet as quickly as possible in a short, choppy fashion as shown. The ankle is held as rigid as possible, and the torso is held upright. Although your legs are moving quickly, your forward motion is relatively slow.

DAN'S TIPS: It helps to visualize the ground as a hot plate, with the balls of your feet reacting to the pain by popping off the "burner."

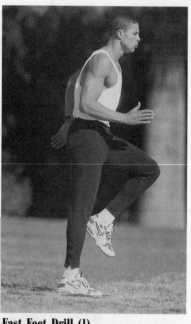

Fast Feet Drill (1)

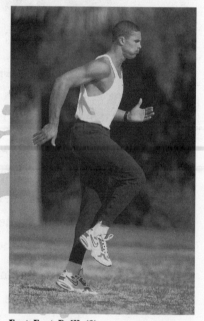

Fast Feet Drill (2)

HIGH KNEES

This drill emphasizes a powerful contraction of the hip flexors and exaggerated extension of the hip. High knees is simply running, but, as shown in the photos, requires taking the front leg through an exaggerated range of motion. Use an alternate arm swing.

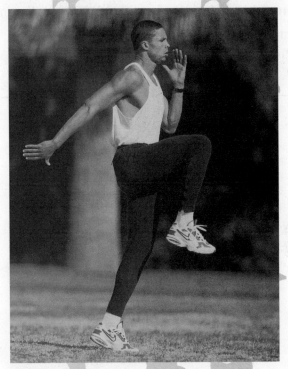

High Knees

DAN'S TIPS: Just as in running and jumping, it's important to maintain an upright posture as you perform this exercise.

SINGLE-LEG BOUNDS

This is an advanced version of double-leg bounds. Stand on one leg with your feet shoulder width apart. Bend your knees, pull your arms back, and jump forward. As you jump, bring both arms forward and in front of you, and then pull them back as you prepare to land on that same leg and jump again. Repeat for the opposite leg.

DAN'S TIPS: Just before you land, hold your breath, and exhale as you jump.

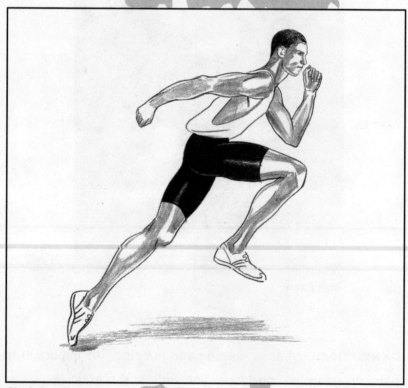

Single-Leg Bounds

SINGLE-LEG HOPS AND SINGLE-LEG HURDLE HOPS

Single-leg hops are performed by simple hopping forward, trying to get the optimal balance between height and distance on each hop to achieve maximum speed. A double-arm pumping action should be used, bringing the arms in front with each hop as shown. Repeat for the other leg. These hops are usually performed for at least 10 yards, with more experienced athletes being able to increase the distance without sacrificing speed.

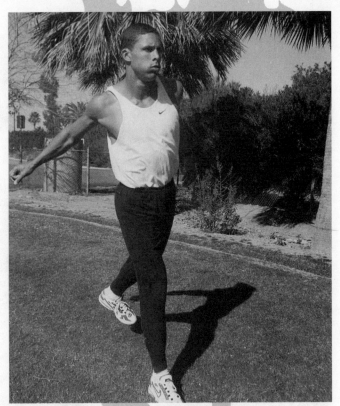

Single-Leg Hops and Single-Leg Hurdle Hops (1)

To perform single-leg hurdle hops, place a series of low hurdles in a row, the height and distance apart of each hurdle based on your jumping ability. Stand in front of the first barrier. Perform the exercise by hopping forward over the hurdles on one leg, swinging your arms back and forth as you do. Repeat for the other leg.

DAN'S TIPS: Arm action is especially important in this exercise to achieve maximum speed. Your arms should be cocked back before you land so that you can spring off the ground quickly.

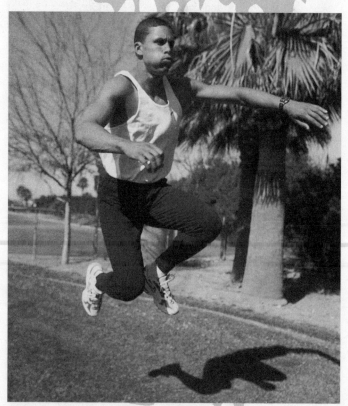

Single-Leg Hops and Single-Leg Hurdle Hops (2)

SKIPPING

This running drill is designed to warm up the knees, calves, and ankles for running and the more intense supplementary drills like bounding. For this drill you skip forward, but use your arms alternately as you would in running.

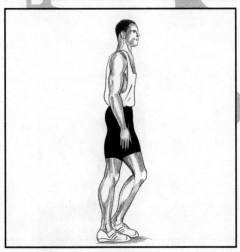

Skipping (1)

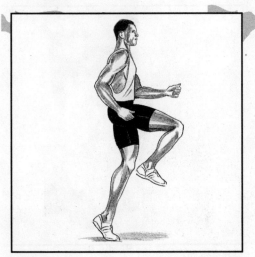

Skipping (2)

Dan's Tips: Because skipping does not require as much effort as bounding exercises, try to focus on running tall and perfecting your arm action.

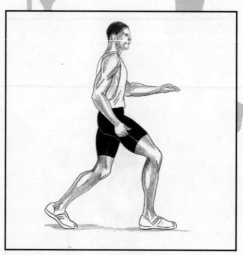

Skipping (3)

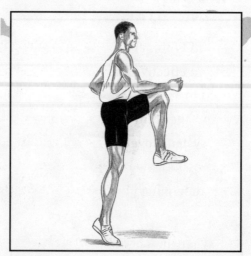

Skipping (4)

COMPONENT FOUR
▲ ENERGY SYSTEM TRAINING

That which doesn't kill you makes you stronger.
                                        —Nietzsche

A man's gotta know his limitations.
                                        —Clint Eastwood

The decathlon demands stamina. Over two days, you continuously push your body to its limits, finishing with the most physically punishing event—the 1500 meters. Such spectacular performance demands both short-term muscular endurance for sprints, jumps, and throws, and long-term cardiovascular endurance to maintain a high energy level throughout the two days of competition.

DEVELOPING STAMINA

It is important to understand the types of energy systems needed to develop an effective endurance program. The first two systems are referred to as oxygen-independent in that they don't require oxygen, and the third energy system is called oxygen-dependent. These systems overlap—you just don't switch from one to another—and the extent to which one is involved in a sporting activity is determined by the intensity and the length of the activity.

The first oxygen-independent energy system is involved in activities of high intensity and short duration. This system is primarily used for movements lasting less than 10 seconds, such as jumps, sprints, and throwing. Football, regardless of the position played, emphasizes this energy system. To train for this type of endurance, work intervals should be less than 30 seconds and rest periods approximately 90 seconds. Thus, a workout that alternates sprinting a half-lap (220 yards) and briskly walking a half-lap targets this energy system.

The second oxygen-independent system is involved in high intensity but slightly longer duration activities. This system becomes the predominant energy system at about 30 seconds into the activity, such as the longer sprints like the 400, and to some extent the 1500. Sports that involve a lot of continuous stop-and-go activity, like basketball and hockey, emphasize this energy system. (In fact, video-tape analysis shows that in a typical basketball game, seldom do the players run as much as a single mile!) To train for this type of endurance, work intervals should be about 30-60 seconds and rest periods approximately 90-180 seconds. Running one lap and briskly walking one lap would mean you are training within this system.

The oxygen-dependent system, which most people like to refer to as the aerobic system, is involved in lower intensity but longer duration activities. This energy system becomes the predominant energy system when an activity continues more than 90 seconds. To train for this type of endurance, work intervals should last about two to three minutes and rest intervals four to six minutes. Running two laps and briskly walking two laps would target this energy system. Because work and rest times are longer, fewer sets are necessary to achieve an optimal training effect.

Many athletes seem to be most concerned about the oxygen dependent system, but this type of conditioning may not be as important as was once thought. Although my workout schedule includes five-mile runs, which in addition to adding variety to my training also develops the mindset to compete in the 1500 meters, I do a minimal amount of long-distance work as it adversely affects the strength component I need to maintain for the other events.

Because performing at the elite level requires seemingly endless hours of training, many athletes can easily become "overtrained" if they perform too much adjunctive long-term endurance work. For instance, with my training schedule it would be counterproductive for me to go to the gym and do an hour on the treadmill or stationary bike. Overtraining reduces an athlete's ability to perform at his or her best and may increase the risk of injury. Therefore, it's important to carefully monitor your workouts to make certain you are not overdoing your endurance work. Again, balance is a key factor in my ultimate workout.

Training for the decathlon is probably the best possible program for exercising a normal, healthy heart. I don't expect (though I may hope) that all of you reading this book are aspiring decathletes. If not, bear in mind that a regular program that includes running, whether short or long distances, makes a healthy heart a stronger and more efficient muscle. Running has been shown to be one of the most effective exercises to protect the heart from disease. Additionally, running will help you better control your weight than other exercise programs.

▲ STARTING OUT

If you presently perform no distance running in your fitness routine, then my advice is to start out slowly. Run on foot-friendly surfaces. Parks are great, not only because they often have groomed dirt trails, but because the environment makes running more pleasurable. Tracks are also excellent because the groomed surface reduces the risk of impact injuries to the feet and ankles, while providing an easily measurable distance.

An important thing to remember about running shoes is that they are for running, not tennis, aerobics, or gardening. This is especially true for activities that require lateral movements, because the high mid-sole of a running shoe makes it unstable. Besides, if you're going to spend a lot of money on running shoes—and trust me, you can spend a *lot* of money on running shoes—then it's wise to prolong their life by using them only for running.

How do you determine which is the best running shoe for you? A good place to start is at a specialty store with employees who know their product. Choose a store with a large inventory so the sales people won't be tempted to put you in a shoe that doesn't fit.

Socks are another important piece of running equipment, and should be purchased when you buy shoes to see how the two products work together. Good socks can provide shock absorption and can help transport perspiration away from the bottom of the feet. Synthetic fibers such as Orlon acrylic and polypropylene are better than cotton fibers—cotton socks cannot transport perspiration away from the feet effectively and often lose their shape when they get wet.

When you begin your run, try to stay on roads that are firm, flat, and smooth. Stay off sidewalks as they are hard and often contain cracks. Grassy areas such as golf courses may contain ruts, and the uneven surface will make you work harder and increase your risk of developing hip, knee, and ankle sprains. The same goes for running on sand at a beach. Local schools often have excellent tracks to run on, but avoid running in only one direction as you could develop muscle imbalances. Avoid indoor tracks if possible, as the banked and frequent turns increase stress on the muscles and joints.

When you run, always breathe through your mouth in order to take in air faster. Breathing through the nose may not supply enough oxygen or thoroughly remove waste products.

Some people who run develop a pain in the side called a "side stitch" by athletes. A side stitch is common in people who are out of shape and training too hard for their current conditioning level. The exact cause of a side stitch is up for debate, but it is probably caused by a lack of oxygen to the diaphragm. Relief from a side stitch can be obtained by reducing your running pace and by concentrating on breathing from the abdominal region instead of the upper chest area.

Drink water as often as possible before, during, and after your runs. Even if you don't feel thirsty, drink water, especially when running in hot or humid conditions. Lack of water may cause heat stroke or cramps.

Heat stroke can be a life-threatening condition and occurs when the body's heat regulating mechanism does not function properly. It is usually caused by rapid fluid loss and excessively high body temperature (104-106 degrees). Muscle cramps are frequently caused by low fluid and potassium levels. To keep your potassium level high, eat lots of fruit. Bananas are an especially good source of potassium.

Unless prescribed by a physician, you should not supplement your diet with excessive salt. High salt levels rob the cells of fluid, thereby increasing your risk of muscle cramps and heat stroke. Again, a lack of fluid is the major cause of heat stroke and muscle cramps, not lack of salt.

▲ INTERVAL TRAINING

Running is hard work. But there is no substitute for endurance training, so dash any hopes for an electrolyte replacement drink or some magical biofeedback electro-stimulus machine to replace this component of fitness. The only way to achieve cardiovascular conditioning is through aerobic work, which is defined as exercise that elevates the heart rate and which continues for at least twenty minutes at a time.

At this point in my career, my training program provides my cardiovascular conditioning. However, if you are not a competitive decathlete but are already a seasoned runner, your running program should probably include interval running.

Interval running is an excellent way to condition your cardiovascular system and decrease your recovery time. This type of training doesn't require you to run at full speed, merely fast enough to bring your pulse up to 180, or about 30 beats in ten seconds. A good rule of thumb for interval training is that you should run six to ten seconds slower than your fastest time for 220 yards with a running start. For most people, this translates into running 220 yards in thirty-two to thirty-five seconds or 440 yards in seventy to seventy-five seconds. As your condition improves, you will need to increase the speed. Recovery should be the time it takes for your pulse to drop to 120 beats per minute, or about 20 beats in ten seconds. This should take about one and one-half minutes, and no more than three.

As your endurance improves you will be able to increase the number of repetitions of the basic distances of 220 and 440 yards. At first you may do as few as ten repetitions, but you should soon increase the number to twenty, thirty, and even forty. You should break them into sets of ten and get a complete rest by walking for five minutes between sets.

Speed interval training is another type of interval training that can be especially helpful for the 1500 meters. It develops the kind of speed-endurance that allows me to sustain a pace close to my top speed for nearly the whole race. Speed interval training is done at racing speed or slightly faster over distances from 110 yards to perhaps as much as 880 yards. The recovery is not as complete as in endurance training because the purpose is to accustom the leg muscles to hard work without complete removal of lactic acid. In this way, the muscles build up a tolerance for continued activity past the point at which you ordinarily would not be able to keep running—an extremely important factor in the tenth event of the decathlon.

In speed interval training, your speed should be three to five seconds slower than your best time for 220 yards with a running start. At first, the recovery interval should consist of walking or jogging until your pulse returns to about 120 beats per minute.

A runner who does endurance interval training by running repeats of 220 yards in thirty-two seconds with a ninety-second recovery interval probably will run speed interval training repeats in twenty-eight to thirty seconds with a recovery interval at first of up to two or three minutes. As you progress, you will want to make the recovery interval shorter. Speed interval training taxes the system much more than regular interval training, and you will find you can't do as many repetitions.

Speed interval training should be used to work on the rhythm of your racing style, and as such may not be appropriate to your individual fitness goals. If, however, you are interested in the decathlon, a series of fast quarter miles will impose a strain something like that encountered in the last part of the 1500. It also helps create a race situation in your mind and then work to keep moving fast and smoothly without tightening up.

▲ SPRINT TRAINING

The last type of running drill I recommend isn't aerobic in nature, but it helps to accustom the cardiovascular system to the demands put on it during a sprint. It's aptly called sprint training and it's one of the best ways to improve your speed. Sprint training requires you to run at or near top speed for short distances of up to 220 yards. The recovery interval is as long as it takes for complete recovery, perhaps as long as five or ten minutes. This allows you to work only on the mechanics of speed.

Sprint training further helps you work on breathing, an essential element to performance. Your breathing, after all, is what is actually feeding your muscles.

Consider this: If you can't negotiate a pair of chopsticks in a traditional Chinese restaurant, you're not going to get much of a meal. The same is true for an athlete who doesn't work on proper breathing—performance will suffer. Just like those chopsticks perform the job of getting food to your mouth, breathing performs the task of getting fuel to your muscles.

I've found that breathing higher—more in the chest than in the diaphragm—changes the adrenaline flow. I use this high breathing to pique my body and hormones so they're prepared for the demands in front of them. I've found that breathing lower calms me down and gets me more into the rhythm. I use this deep breathing technique for the long events, particularly the 1500, where I find it also helps to numb the pain.

Whether your schedule allows you to devote two hours or ten hours a week to running, it is an essential component to the ultimate workout. Find the time, do the task, and you will reap the benefits.

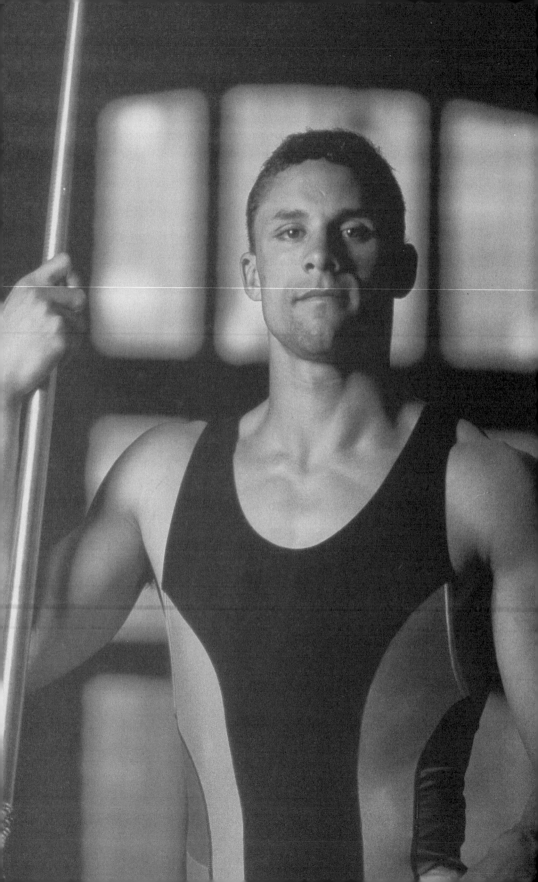

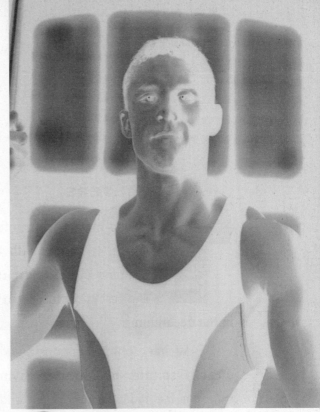

THE SPORT
OF DECATHLON

▲ 100 METERS

The 100 meters is an intense, straight-ahead sprint. It begins with the athlete virtually jumping out of the starting blocks. It is the shortest sprinting event at the Olympics and in the decathlon.

Michael Johnson is considered by many to be the greatest sprinter of all time, having run phenomenal times in the 1996 Olympic 200- and 400-meter events. However, the title of "Fastest Man in the World" traditionally has gone to the world record holder or the Olympic champion in the 100 meters. Using this barometer, that title must rightfully go to Donovan Bailey, a Canadian who was born in Jamaica. Bailey broke the world record in 9.84 seconds while winning the gold medal in the Atlanta Games. Fellow Canadian Ben Johnson has run faster in Olympic competition, but his records and gold medal were rescinded when he tested positive for steroids at the 1988 Olympics.

A major change in the 100-meter event occurred when automatic, electronic timing replaced manual timing. It is surprising that hand-timed races tended to make the athletes seem faster than they actually were. For example, from June 20, 1968 through May 22, 1976, nine sprinters ran the 100 meters in 9.9, equaling the world record. But it wasn't until June 14, 1991 that Leroy Burrell of the United States was able to match this time in an electronically timed race.

Because many football coaches still use handheld stopwatches, track athletes tend to be rather skeptical when we hear about all those "4.2-second, 40-yard dashes" claimed by football players. And, just because an athlete is fast for 40 yards doesn't mean he can maintain that speed for 100 meters. During the race when Carl Lewis broke the world record, Leroy Burrell held the lead until the last ten meters. Also, many throwers and weightlifters can hold their own with elite sprinters for the first twenty meters. Shotputter Brian Oldfield, who weighed about 275 pounds, often gave exhibitions in which he would race the best female sprinters for short distances—races he usually won.

Two factors that can better running times are high altitude and tailwinds, although there is a restriction as to how much wind speed is permitted to establish a world record. Although you can't predict exactly what the wind speed will be during a race, or for that matter which direction it's blowing, you can often choose where to run. The first official world record with electronic timing was recorded by James Hines at the Mexico City Olympics (7300-feet elevation) in 1968, and Calvin Smith broke that record fifteen years later in Colorado Springs (6000 feet). Although the higher elevation will help the sprinting and jumping events, the air is thinner at higher altitudes, making it extremely difficult to run the 1500—or for that matter get through an entire decathlon.

The 100 meters is one of my best events, and it's the first event of the decathlon. If you get a good start on the 100, you'll most likely have a good decathlon. The same holds true if you get a bad start—you'll be fighting an uphill battle the entire way to try to finish at the top. (For the record, the worst start in a decathlon belonged to West Germany's Jurgen Hingsen. Hingsen, who broke the world record for the decathlon three times and had a best result of 8832 points, was a heavy favorite to win the 1988 Olympics in Seoul, but was disqualified for false starting in the 100 meters.)

My favorite 100-meter race came in 1991. That was the year I qualified for my first World Championships. I ran it in 10.22. I don't really remember the gun going off—I just remember a bang as I blasted off. The race was over before I knew it.

I can usually tell before a race how I'm going to run it. If I feel tight—tense, too anxious, stiff—then I know it's not going to be good. Picture in your mind the way a race horse stretches to finish just a split second ahead. That's the way you need to feel at the start of a 100-meter race—as if you could stretch your neck out and put it right over the finish line. That's why I always make certain I get a good warm-up, and also get myself psyched to give it my all. When I get in position at the start line, there is only one thought in my mind: *Quick, quick, quick.* That's the essence of the 100 meters.

The 100 meters is a rhythm race; it's all tempos and technique. If you want to know how the 100 meters should be run, watch Carl Lewis. He runs it upright, relaxed, and his arms move in a perfect pumping motion—there is no wasted energy. As for myself, I've always had a good 100 meters because I'm a natural sprinter. I have great speed because I can harness intensity at the start of the race—harness it, and then channel it.

To run a good 100 you need to be able to *explode* out of the starting blocks, and for this you need ballistic strength. Coach Sloan says that I've got more ballistic strength than anyone he's ever seen. My mom says that when I was a child, I'd jump off the couch and pop right up into a run before she had her head turned. My mom wasn't thrilled, but it was an early sign of ballistic strength potential.

When you're in good enough shape to run the 100, the 400, the half-mile or the mile, it's a great feeling—it feels as if you can start sprinting and run forever. You feel like you'll never get fatigued. When you start thinking about your running instead of just feeling that freedom, that's when your run will start to fall apart.

Training for the 100, 400, and even the 1500 is key to a decathlete, and when it comes to running, I tell people, "You have to live it." People think of sprinters as just being fast, natural runners. Genetics is important, but you have to train to be fast, and you have to train for endurance. The more you can train, and the more you give of yourself, the better off you'll be.

▲ LONG JUMP

Unlike the broad jump, which begins from a stationary position, the long jump begins with a sprint to a takeoff board followed by a jump into a sand pit. The closest impression in the sand to the takeoff board, by any part of the jumper's body, determines the length of the jump. Because the speed of the sprint is a primary determinant of the final result, athletes who can run fast often excel in this event.

Carl Lewis, a four-time gold medal winner at the Olympics, is considered one of the best in the long jump, even though he never captured the world record. Two other notables in this event are the legendary Jesse Owens, who held the world record for more than 25 years, and Bob Beamon, who held it for more than 22 years until Mike Powell exceeded it in 1991 with a mark of 29 feet, 4 1/2 inches. A silver medalist in 1992, Powell almost didn't make the trip to the Atlanta Olympics, needing all his attempts at the trials to just qualify for the team. He settled down at the games, however, and came home with his second silver medal.

Like the sprints, high altitude helps long jump performance. Bob Beamon's record, which smashed the previous standard of 27 feet, 4 3/4 inches, occurred at an altitude of 7,300 feet in Mexico City. Interestingly, after achieving his record of 29 feet, 2 1/2 inches, Beamon couldn't come within two feet of that record. Carl Lewis was thought to be the first athlete who would break Beamon's remarkable world record, having consistently jumped over 28 feet in major competitions. Lewis refused to seek out competitions held at high altitude (not to mention dividing his focus on the sprints) and he never achieved a record. However, the payoff for such diversity was a treasure chest of gold medals and a place in history as one of the greatest track athletes of all time.

A great long jump feels like someone has connected a rope to the top of your head and just pulls you off the platform, up into the air, and right into the pit. It's like one clean movement designed to propel an object as far as possible. It's effortless.

The long jump is one of my best events. I've been working at it since junior high school. I was fast, and a good jumper. That's all you need. I'm still number two at the University of Idaho in the long jump.

My best long jump performance was in Talence, France, when I broke the record with 26 feet, 9 inches. My worst jumps were at Atlanta. During 1996, I'd changed my technique. Even though we had the best intentions, the method I was using didn't give me the best landing.

In the long jump, you have two options: the hitch kick or the hang technique. Carl Lewis does a hitch kick. He leaves the ground and pretends as if he is running in the air until he lands. The hang technique is when you jump and let your legs hang, and then at the very end you kick your legs out and land. I do a combination, a hitch-hang. I'll take off and do a hitch for a half-cycle, then I'll bring my legs together in a hang and kick them out at the end. Last year I tried a complete hitch where I ran all the way to my landing. It may work for Carl, but I wasn't hitting the sand very well.

When it comes to getting off the board in the long jump, you can't beat work in the weight room. An increase in the amount of weight you're working with on the squat and power clean translates directly to more power off the board. An explosive exercise such as the power clean is excellent in this regard, as are basic strength moves like the squat.

Timing on the approach is important. If you *miss the board* (landing on or over it before you jump) you don't score, and if you jump too soon you lose distance. Carl Lewis, in the jump that won him the gold medal in the 1992 Olympics, took off about a foot behind the boards—had he been closer he might have broken the world record. It's also essential during the approach to accelerate quickly and achieve good sprinting form, keeping the chin up and lifting the rib cage. Because of the importance of the approach, I practice it quite a bit. I practice it two to three days a week for an hour.

Finally, landing technique is very important to achieve a good mark on the long jump. If you land on your butt, you're giving up all the inches between your feet and your butt. If you land where your feet are, then you're going to get six, eight inches or even a foot farther. The hitch got me off the board better, but my landings were horrible. Coach Sloan and I realized it right before Olympics, so I went back to my old technique—running fast right until I reached the end, then kicking out my legs.

▲ SHOT PUT

The shot is a brass or iron ball that weighs sixteen pounds. The athlete stands in the middle of a circle that is seven feet in diameter, and assumes the starting position by resting the ball on his shoulder. Without leaving the circle, the athlete either spins or glides across the rink and "puts" the ball (as opposed to "throwing" it) as far as possible. The longest distance achieved determines the winner.

Because there is a relationship between size, strength, and the ability to put the shot, it's not uncommon to see men weighing over three hundred pounds compete in this event. One exception was Al Feuerbach of the United States, who won the USA Weightlifting National Championships in the 242-pound weight class and broke the world record in the shot put in 1973. Of course, carrying a large amount of body weight would severely limit my performance in my other events, so I make a compromise in body weight when it comes to this event.

The United States has pretty much dominated this event in international competition. The Russians, known for their big men in weightlifting, have always been competitive in this event, but their last world record holder was Aleksandr Baryshnikov, who threw 72 feet, 2 1/4 inches in 1976.

Baryshnikov was considered responsible for introducing, or at least popularizing, the rotational technique of throwing the shot. In contrast to the gliding style in which the athlete essentially hops in a straight line to the edge of the circle, the rotational style has the athlete spinning around the rink. The glide style is still used by some athletes, especially beginners, because it is easier to learn and because some athletes simply perform better with it.

In the open shot put competition, each athlete is allowed six attempts, but most often the best throws are achieved during the first three attempts. One notable exception was Alessandro Andrei of Italy, who on August 12, 1987, set world records in his final three attempts with 74 feet, 6 1/2 inches, 74 feet, 11 1/4 inches, and 75 feet, 2 inches. (Although Andrei was considered the first man to officially throw 75 feet, in 1975 Brian Oldfield of the United States threw 75 feet as a professional.)

The shot put is an event where people think I'm going to be weak because I don't have enough strength. United States Olympian Richard Marks could snatch 375 pounds, and the Eastern Bloc had some enormously strong throwers, including a female who could supposedly bench press 440 pounds. Sure, high levels of strength and a heavier body weight provide an advantage that translates into about fifteen feet greater distance, but this event is really about technique. It's about getting into the correct body position and using your legs.

Coach Sloan and I don't even look to the heavyweight shot-putters because it's our opinion that few of them have what we would consider optimal technique—they use their body weight to muscle the shot without finessing it. They would be great examples if I wanted to bring my body weight up to three hundred pounds—but since that's not the case, I rely on my coaches for inspiration in the shot.

My best experience in the shot was in Talence, France, when I broke the record in 1992. In 1995, I struggled with the shot because I forgot the basics. Looking back, I believe that in our search for something new, we went to the advanced level and got too technical, ignoring the very basics of throwing the shot. Often in track, you may go overboard with technical details and become confused. The expression "paralysis by analysis" sums up the problem.

Unlike the 100 meters and the long jump, the shot put is an event I only began doing to compete in the decathlon. It wasn't one of my sports of choice. Still, I intrinsically understand how to use my body to create power. Like golf and a dozen other sports I've played, I got off to a really great start, immediately performing at an adequate proficiency—but then I leveled off. At that point, I believe that's the sign that you need to move on to a better coach, or a sport-specific coach, to show you some new techniques. Coach Sloan is a field events specialist, and I've been quite lucky that when I've reached these plateaus I haven't had to search much further.

The shot put is driven by torque from your torso, which means your abdominals and legs have to be in great shape to power the motion. Your arms are there as levers, not sources of power. The power starts in your legs, pummels upwards into the torso, then moves up into the shoulders, which effectively release the weight like a slingshot.

When you throw a good shot, you can actually feel the power transferring from your legs through your torso and right to the tips of your fingers, like a giant unwinding top. In the final moments, you can feel your fingers actually flip the shot as it leaves your body's catapult. Incidentally, the chalk that seems to get all over the faces of shot putters as they compete and practice helps their technique because it enables them to securely hold the ball and prevents it from slipping off their shoulders.

Good posture is essential to the shot, as it enables you to get into the best position to apply your power. It's also important not to *rush* the shot. An athlete who hurries the throw is one who doesn't put any body into the throw, then tries to push it with his arms. It is important in the shot to finish with all your power. I like to draw the analogy from the martial arts, where the master tells you to try to punch *through* the board, not *to* it. It's the same with the shot and discus: You need to finish completely past the point of your release.

Once you've learned the basic technique of throwing the shot, my best advice to you is to stick with it. Practice. Be consistent. Then, when the technique has become second nature to you, work on your intensity. Think of yourself as a top that has to become physically and mentally wound up. The big Olympic weightlifters and shot-putters are usually the ones to scream and stomp at the end of an event. But if you look back at me and at other decathletes, you'll see the same face contorted with a scream at the end of the shot. It's the only way to release the intensity you have to muster to master this event.

▲ HIGH JUMP

In the high jump event, the athlete takes a running start and, jumping off one foot, leaps over a bar resting between a set of supports. If the athlete clears the bar without it falling, the attempt is considered good. You have three attempts at each height you choose, you must always increase the height, and you can pass on any height. Your best successful result is considered your final mark. Because you are given three attempts at each height you choose, the high jump can be one of the longest events.

In the early days of the high jump, most athletes used the "scissors" style, in which they straddled the bar. Although it is still used, the most popular style was invented by Dick Fosbury of the United States, who won the gold medal with his "flop" technique at the 1968 Olympics. In this style, the athlete jumps with his back to the bar; this puts him in a better posture to transfer his center of gravity over the bar.

Most people don't realize it, but the world record in this event is over eight feet. The first and only athlete to reach this height is Javier Sotomayor of Cuba who achieved the mark on July 29, 1989. Because of his persistence, Sotomayor was able to establish his next world record four years later with a mark of 8 feet 1/2 inch. An improvement of a half-inch may not seem like much progress, but he was the best ever at the event. And with the exception of phenoms, like Michael Johnson, who make the track and field statisticians shake their heads in wonder, improvements in world records most often are made in the smallest increments.

Interestingly, if the athletes were allowed to jump off both feet, the records in this event might be much higher. For example, in 1954, Dick Browing, a tumbler from the United States, was reported to have performed a somersault over a bar set at 7 feet 6 inches. In fact, in the '60s, several long jumpers were experimenting with trying to perform somersaults during their event, and in practice, a few in fact came surprisingly close to the world record. The track and field federation, however, decided not to allow this technique to be used in competition, most likely because it posed a great risk of permanent neck injury.

My best experience in the high jump came in 1994 at the Goodwill Games. That was the year that Dwight Stones, a world-renowned high jumper (and the last American to hold the world record in this event) who was commentating the event, came up to me beforehand and commented on the hard surface. "You'll be lucky if you jump six-ten today," he said. It was true, we were on a hard, tight surface, which makes it very difficult to run at high speed. The track I train on at Washington State isn't so tight; you can actually feel your spikes go into the track. But in 1994 the track felt like concrete. Still, I had a lot of respect for Dwight Stones. He was the first guy to clear seven feet from both the right and left sides and to straddle it. When I heard his challenge, I vowed to prove him wrong. Well, that's putting it mildly. I said to myself, "Bull. I'll show you."

That day I jumped 7 feet, 2 1/2 inches.

The high jump is a particularly challenging event because you have to stay continually motivated to jump higher. It's an event you have to always work at. You rarely see gains in a short period of time—it sometimes takes years to achieve a new personal best. Also, being able to jump high from a standing position does not necessarily mean you can automatically be a great high jumper, as evidenced by the fact that discus throwers and weightlifters often can jump higher from standing than top high jumpers. Weighing well over three hundred pounds, the great super heavyweight weightlifter Vassily Alexeyev was reported to have high jumped over six feet, and American weightlifter Mark Henry, weighing over 400 pounds, could dunk a basketball. Of course, not all high jumpers have a problem jumping from a standing position—former world record holder Valery Brumel from Russia could kick a basketball rim.

The key to a successful high jump is the approach to the bar. You run forward for four strides, lean to the front standard for two, work to the far standard for four, then take off. It involves a lot of technique to create the necessary force that you need through the corner to generate the upward momentum for takeoff.

The high jump is very hard on the body. I've seen pictures in which it looks like the bone in my takeoff leg is bending when I plant my foot. But even though the biomechanics of the takeoff aren't entirely natural, the overall *feel* of the high jump is. And for me it's actually a fun event because it draws upon track and field components that I'm good at: leg strength, bounding ability, and most importantly, intensity.

I practice the high jump for one hour, two times a week. Nearly all my field-event training is done in a group, which simulates the feeling of a competition. It also means that during an hour I may jump fifteen to twenty times, not the thirty or more times I would if I were training on my own.

The success I've had with the high jump has largely come from my ability to avoid injuries. It's a fact that high jump medals have been won not so much by stellar performances, but by an athlete's ability to avoid the injuries that permeate this event. For me, as soon as I feel run-down, I take a break. This may frustrate my coaches, but I'd rather miss a few workouts and be fit, healthy, and one hundred percent than make the workouts and be slightly injured.

The biggest mistake an athlete can make on the high jump is to try to jump the bar. Like the shot put and pole vault, a lot of things take place on the ground first. Proper technique occurs at the point of takeoff—it doesn't occur when you're in the air trying to go over the bar. That's the misconception young kids have. As soon as I leave the ground, I'm vulnerable to whatever I did during and up to the takeoff. I can't do much in the air to help save or make a jump.

My personal training goal is to be consistent—to be a 7-foot consistent high jumper. For me, the high jump is still a hot and cold event.

▲ 400 METERS

Many people believe that 400 meters is four laps around the track. Close, but the 400-meter event is actually 2.34 meters longer than that. In the past, many athletes considered this event a run, but with the quality of today's athletes, the 400 meters is considered a sprint in which athletes approach the same speeds attained in the 100 meters. In the decathlon, the 400 meters is the last event of the first day of competition, and you want to perform well to finish on a high note.

The world record is held by Harry "Butch" Reynolds of the United States, who in 1990 faced a two-year ban for allegedly failing a drug test. He sued the International Amateur Athletic Federation (IAAF), claiming that there were irregularities in the testing. He won 27.3 million dollars and was eventually allowed to compete again. He made the 1996 Olympic team but withdrew in the semifinals due to injury.

Reynolds may be the world record holder in this event, but the most famous athlete in the 400 meters is Michael Johnson. Johnson, the world record holder in the 200 meters with a time of 19.32, competes in both events at international competitions, a particularly difficult accomplishment because of all the qualifying rounds that must be completed. Nevertheless, in Atlanta he not only competed in both the 200 and the 400, but in the process shattered his own world record in the 200 meters and set an Olympic record of 43.49 in the 400.

What's also interesting about this event is that thanks to Johnson's popularity and intense lobbying, he convinced the IAAF to adjust the qualifying schedules of the 200- and 400-meter races so that he would be better able to perform in both events. This is unprecedented in track and field. (In the movie *Chariots of Fire*, Eric Liddell, 400-meter Olympic Champion in 1924, supposedly withdrew from the 100 meters because the heats would be run on a Sunday, which would conflict with his religious beliefs. Emotional appeals from the British coaches failed to change the schedule, but in a remarkable example of sportsmanship, teammate Lord Burghley gave Liddell his spot on the 400. Although it made for a great story, in real life Liddell knew about the schedule more than six months before the race, not as he was boarding the boat to Paris, and apparently Burghley wasn't even on the team for the 400.)

My best experience was in 1991 at the Tokyo World Championships. I was up against guys who had personal bests better than mine. That day I ran 46.5 and far surpassed everyone in the race. That event made me a world champion, and it didn't matter to me what I did on the second day. Before the race I was the most nervous I've ever been. But after the gun went off I didn't feel any pain; I just dug in deep until the end. I was "in the zone" for that race. The two outdoor 400 meters at the 1996 Olympic trials and games were also memorable for me because they were both fast races. I knew I was in great shape and ready to give it my all.

Michael Johnson says he likes the 400 because there's more room for mistakes; and that translates into more room for perfection. The 400 to me is the biggest gut-check out there. I'm more concerned about the 400 than I'll ever be about the 1500.

Running the 400 is a sprint that you hold on to as long as you can. To do that you need to find a pace that is both comfortable and uncomfortable. You can't sprint full out; you've got to back it off just a little bit. Mentally, the 400 is the event that makes or breaks a decathlete. It's an event where you break through barriers—in training and in competition. You learn to feel every step, think every step, and develop ultimate control over all aspects of the race.

Pain is part of the 400. You need to control fear in this event because if you've trained for it properly, you know it is going to hurt. No matter how fast or slow you run, it always hurts. You reach a point where you accept this pain, and since either way you go it's going to hurt, you might as well give it your all. I've only had a few bad experiences with this event, and those times were when I questioned my fitness and training. My personal goals are to get mentally tougher by realizing that my body can withstand the punishment I put it through, and by reminding myself that it only hurts for a little while.

Training for the 400 takes about three workouts a week. It's the same kind of training as the 100 and 200; the only difference is your start. I work hardest on the 400. I believe if you can run the 400, then you can run the 200 and 100 much more effectively.

The 400 is an event that you have to be in shape for. When you are, you know it. There will be a bounce in your stride. You'll run up stairs without getting tired. It's a real core part of decathlon training. If you're in 400-meter shape, you're in decathlon shape.

▲ 110-METER HIGH HURDLES

In the 110-meter high hurdles, each athlete sprints 110 meters while clearing ten hurdles that are 3 feet, six inches high. Each hurdle is shaped in an inverted *T*, which easily falls over, so as to reduce the possibility of injury to the athlete.

The 110-meter high hurdles event has traditionally been dominated by Americans, with eighteen of the past twenty-five world record holders being United States citizens. One of the most versatile athletes was Willie Davenport, world record holder in 1969. Davenport used his speed to compete in the four-man bobsled in the 1980 Olympics. Likewise, Edwin Moses, former world record holder in

400-meter hurdles, was a member of the 1990 and 1991 United States World Cup bobsled teams.

Football coaches often look for 100-meter sprinters to play in the skill positions. Bob Hayes (world record holder in 1964) played with the 1971 Superbowl Champion Dallas Cowboys, James Hines (three-time world record holder, once in 1967 and twice in 1968) played with the Miami Dolphins. Even more important, hurdlers may be good choices for football because they have to react to contact and be able to make lightning-quick adjustments in their stride as they run.

My best hurdles ever came at the Bruce Jenner Classic in 1994 in San Jose, California. I finished in 13.44, second in the race but my fastest time ever. Looking back at some of my best races, it's not always the first-place finishes that stand out, or even the personal bests. In this case it was just a feeling I had. I crossed the line and felt good inside about it. I had run that race with reckless abandon—I even thought I was going to fall down a couple of times. That's the feeling that sticks with me.

The hurdles has always been my mainstay event and an excellent event with which to begin my second day of the decathlon. I started winning them as a high school junior, and not much has changed. At first I didn't train much; I just went out and won the hurdles every time.

The hurdles is the event that was the easiest for me to learn, and for which I am probably the most gifted. The first time I ran them I was a sophomore in high school. I was getting ready to do my first decathlon ever, just for fun. My coach said, "You're going to have to run hurdles," so off I went. My first time out I ran it right and I ran it fast. From that day forward I've always thought of the hurdles as my event.

I advanced in the hurdles fast. In high school I had a lot of breakthrough races. I'd run fifteen seconds, then the next weekend I'd do fourteen. Then, as a senior, I broke into the thirteens. You plateau for a while, then one race you're more relaxed, things come together, and you have a breakthrough.

The hurdles are nothing more than a sprint—you just have to learn how to sprint over the hurdles. Flexibility is important, as is balance. More important than those two is aggressiveness. You have to be very aggressive and not afraid to bang your knee or fall down. I've never fallen in a race, but I've done my share in practice. That's just part of the event.

Concentration is critical in hurdling. You need to be able to focus one hundred percent on your race. When you're running the hurdles, there is movement all around you and there is a lot of pushing and shoving—each lane is only 45 inches wide. You may get hit, or someone might slap you with their trail arm. There's a lot of distraction, but you have to stay focused. If you look at Carl Lewis in 1988 against Ben Johnson, you see him looking around to see where everyone else is. That may have cost him the race. Greg Foster used to win because he hit the guy next to him in the chest about five times; that's going to slow anyone down.

One of my theories on the hurdles is that if you're out in front, no one can hit you. Still, you can't let go of your race. Because you're out ahead, you can bet that there is someone right behind you doing all he can to take you from behind.

Height plays a role in the hurdles. If you're too tall you have to cut your stride. If you're too short you'll have trouble getting over the hurdles. Me—I'm about the right height, but I think the best hurdler of all time was Renaldo Nehemiah. He was the perfect height, and to watch him hurdle was to see poetry in motion.

The biggest thing that can go wrong in the hurdles is something called *pressing*—you force your run, you try to catch somebody, you grit your teeth. Relaxation is definitely the key. I've seen many people trip and fall because they were pressing, trying to get over the hurdle too fast instead of trying to run fast and stay relaxed.

I practice the hurdles three times a week, and as with all the track events, posture and rhythm are very important. In the hurdles, it's about turning over your stride. You want to keep your stride light and tall—not forced. You can actually hear a good hurdling stride: *voomp, voomp, voomp.* You need to think it, feel it, hear it, then you are in control of it.

Edwin Moses talked a lot about the high hurdles. In particular, he talked about how so many people look at them as a barrier, something to be feared and then conquered. Edwin was unique in that he saw the hurdles as a barrier, but a barrier that he could place between himself and the other competitors. That's the way I run the hurdles. The 110-meter high hurdles is an event that lets me put distance between myself and my opponents. It's not an obstacle in the decathlon, but a helpmate.

▲ DISCUS

The discus weighs four pounds, seven ounces, and, like the shot, is thrown from a circle, although slightly larger with a diameter of 8 feet, 2 1/2 inches. The athlete is given six attempts, and the best distance achieved without the athlete stepping out of the circle is recorded as the best result.

When you think of the Olympics and track and field, the first event that comes to many people's minds is the discus. The statue *Discobolus*, which shows an athlete preparing to throw the discus, is a pose that is often copied to represent the Olympic Games and the sport of track and field.

What *Discobolus* is to sculpture, Al Oerter is to the discus. A four-time gold medalist and four-time world record holder in this event, he was also credited with being the first man to break the two-hundred-foot barrier. His best throw came in 1980 at age forty-three, when he threw 227 feet, 10 3/4 inches. Also of note are John Powell, world record holder in 1975, and Mac Wilkins, who broke the world record four times in 1976. These two had epic battles. Although Wilkins upstaged Powell in 1976 by taking the gold and again in 1984 when he took second to Powell's third, Powell finished his career with the longest throw at the 1987 World Championships, 236 feet, 6 inches, at the age of forty.

Wind is a factor in this event as a headwind increases the lift of the discus. The current record of 243 feet was established in 1986 by Jurgen Schult. It was reported that a strong headwind helped the flight of this discus, a report that may be true when you consider his best throw since then is 231 feet, 2 inches. Considering that only two men have managed to exceed seventy meters, or about 230 feet in this decade, the present record is likely to stand for some time.

When I think of the discus and my best moment, I think back to Boise, 1992. That would have to have been my perfect discus throw. I was like a top unwinding, in perfect balance, using my levers to increase the spin and getting the maximum stretch-reflex action. My left arm opened up my chest, showing my chest to the field, then I pulled my left arm back, stretching my whole right side. I felt as if my left leg was a hinge on a gate and I was swinging my entire body around it. I knew the throw was good—it had to be to feel that perfect. I hit 174 feet that day, my best ever.

The discus was one of the events I learned for the decathlon, and it was easy for me to reach a proficient level. I presently train in the discus twice a week to increase my power and stay on my balance while doing it.

Today, I approach my training from a conservative standpoint. But back in junior college I was much more of an extremist, particularly in events like the discus and shot. I remember putting a towel out at 150 feet and taking fifty throws using good release and good technique, trying to hit that towel. Then I'd head inside and do standing throws, where you're not turning.

My breakthrough in the discus came as most breakthroughs do: from my coach. I was putting in the time practicing, but my technique just wasn't working. The only saving grace was that even though my posture was bad coming out of the back, when it came time to throw I would find a way to get into the right position. My coach showed me how to be in the right position coming out of the back, and the whole throw went better. I learned to really control my movements and focus on different cues. That's an important lesson in the discus. As with a driver in golf, you need to practice, practice, practice. And when you do it enough times, all of a sudden it feels easy and just comes naturally.

The discus can't be rushed. Good posture is important, but the most critical element is tempo. You're turning twice, and the turns have to be the same—in perfect tempo and rhythm. That's what you need to work on. You also need to listen to the way you sound. *Voom, voom*—that's the sound of a good discus throw.

▲ POLE VAULT

As in the high jump, in pole vault competition the athlete takes a running start and jumps, or rather vaults, over a bar set on supports. If the athlete clears the bar without it falling, the attempt is considered good. And, like the high jump, the athlete has three attempts at each height chosen, must always increase the height, and can pass on any height. Your best successful result is considered your final mark. Because you are given three attempts at each height, it takes considerable time to set up the support. The pole vault is also one of the longest events; often, with enough competitors, you'll see this event starting in the morning and ending in the evening.

The pole vault pits have changed from sawdust on level sand to foam, allowing vaulters to land more safely. Wind is a factor in this event, and the ideal condition is zero—which is why some vaulters prefer the indoor season. Wind or no wind, pole vaulters are considered the daredevils of track and field.

The materials used to make poles have varied over the years, including everything from bamboo to fiberglass, which, because of its springiness, requires a high degree of skill to master. One of the first to use these poles was Bob Seagren, who won the gold medal in this event in 1968. Unfortunately, when the fiberglass pole he brought to the 1972 games was banned, the best he could do with the old-style poles (which he hadn't been practicing with) was the silver medal. Later on, fiberglass poles were allowed, but the whole incident left a bad taste in Seagren's mouth. Seagren went on to win the Superstars competition in 1973, which pitted top athletes against each other in unfamiliar sports. Seagren's victory gave those unfamiliar with track and field a greater respect for the athleticism of track athletes.

The king of the pole vault in the modern era is unquestionably Sergei Bubka of Russia. Bubka's first record was set in 1984 with 19 feet, 2 1/2 inches, and he went on to break that record 16 times! He finished with an incredible vault of 20 feet, 1 3/4 inches in 1994, and is still the only vaulter to clear the twenty-foot barrier. His textbook-perfect technique, great pound-for-pound strength, and overall athleticism and scientific approach to training make Bubka the role model for this event.

One of the best decathletes of his era was Yang Chuan-Kwang of Taiwan, a world record holder in 1963 with 8009 points, which included a personal best of 15 feet, 10 1/2 inches in the pole vault. At the time, this vault was about seven inches away from the world record, and was above the highest accounted score in the charts that determine the point total.

The pole vault is an event that I wasn't very good at for a long time—and I'm not talking about the no-heighter. That remains a fluke in my career that I can't exactly explain. It just happened, and since then I've made certain all the elements within my control are in control, to keep it from ever repeating.

The pole vault takes guts—pure guts. People who don't pole vault can't imagine running full out with a sixteen-foot pole and then planting one end while you hold on to the other. But to do the pole vault well, you can't have any fear. For me, that took some time. Back in high school I had a pole break on me (a problem that will not happen with today's poles), and I didn't vault for a while after that experience.

When I got back into vaulting, I was still plagued by doubt. My worst years were 1988, 1989 and 1990—every time I got to the pole vault I would worry. At the Goodwill Games in 1990 I only did thirteen feet—Dave Johnson did seventeen feet, took the lead, and beat me. That experience may have been what made me finally say, "No more." I was not going to let the pole vault beat me, and that's when I started vaulting better and with more consistency.

My best moments in the pole vault came in all three of the World Championships. I vaulted seventeen feet and had good attempts. You get your best pole vault when there is no wind; weather can have a tremendous influence when you're trying to put this sixteen-foot pole into a little eighteen-inch box. If the wind blows too hard from right to left, you can't judge exactly where the tip of the pole is going to go. If you have wind in your face, it upsets your step. Your step placement is very important. The place you take that last step has to be timed perfectly with your hand position. If the wind is at your back it can be a disaster. Like the long jump, the pole vault is about a nice consistent run, every time. If you blow that, it can be a disaster—and disaster in the vault usually means injury. I can't tell you how many times I've left the ground and said, "uh-oh!"

I sometimes use the analogy of a kid's bicycle jump. You take a board and angle it up with bricks. If you hit the board fast, you're going to fly—but if you hit it too slow, your front tire is going to get stuck. That's how the pole vault is. You can't "kind of" do the pole vault. You have to go for it or you're going to hurt yourself. Athletes who are protective in the pole vault are the ones that land on their heads. You have to let yourself go, just like in the high jump. Those are the two events where I say to myself, "Let it go. Let the run go, then let it fly."

Tall athletes have an advantage in the pole vault. Picture the tip of the pole in the box at takeoff. The taller you are, the less angle you will have to create. That angle is what establishes your takeoff. When you make that plant, you need to get your hands up as high overhead as possible. The Russians do this extremely well.

The pole vault is less injurious today because of the quality of the poles. I use poles of different flexes. For training, I use poles twenty pounds heavier than I should be jumping on. It's an exciting day when you have a breakthrough and you can get on a longer pole, which will shoot you higher in the air, or use a pole with stiffer flex to give you more spring.

The most critical part of the vault is the plant. I train in the pole vault twice a week, and when I'm running down the runway, my coach is right there with me yelling, "Tip up! Keep the tip up! Now—take off!" Everyone wants to get over that bar, but you can't get over the bar if you don't take off right.

When I was correcting my bad technique, I vaulted almost every day for a year with Coach Sloan. Now I'm back to Tuesdays and Thursdays, and I'm still working on eliminating little bad habits that keep me from jumping extremely high. I hold back a little. I don't quite let myself plant the pole as effectively as I should. The bad habits have created a bad left arm, and I don't let myself fly away like I should, especially when I have the wind in my face. I'm working at those things, though. That's what being a world champion is all about.

▲ JAVELIN

The javelin is made of metal, although originally made of wood, and is thrown after a short run. Each competitor is given six attempts, and the best throw (measured by the furthest tip of the javelin) determines the winner.

Like the discus, the javelin is another event with its roots in the ancient Olympics, and its aesthetic appeal makes it a model event for the games. The sport has been dominated by Europeans in the modern era, with the exception of Tom Petranoff of the United States, who broke the world record in 1983. One decathlete, Aleksander Klumberg of Estonia, who broke the world record in 1922 with 6087 points, competed in both the javelin and decathlon in the 1920 and 1924 Olympics. His best Olympic result was a bronze in the decathlon and fifth in the javelin. His throw of 62.20 meters was the best decathlon score for 30 years.

One of the greatest javelin throwers was Matti Jarvinen of Finland, who broke ten world records, his first being 234 feet, 9 inches in 1930 and his last being 253 feet, 4 inches in 1936. His brother, Akilles, became a world record holder in the decathlon, with 6,865 points in 1930, and won two silver medals in the Olympic Games, 1928 and 1932.

Because of a fear that the distance of the throws might injure spectators or other athletes on the field, after six-foot-six inch Uwe Hohn of Germany threw 343 feet, 10 inches in 1984, the balance of the javelin was changed in 1986 to a different center of gravity to minimize this risk. The first record with this new javelin was set by Klaus Tafelmeier of France, with a throw of 282 feet, 3 inches on September 21, 1986, but seven world records later, the best mark is 323 feet,

1 inch by Jan Zelezny of Czechoslovakia, made on May 25, 1996. Hohn suffered a back injury in 1986 at age twenty-four, and was no longer able to throw and see what he would have done with the new javelin.

The javelin was one of the most difficult events for me to learn. The problem is that I'm a thrower—I love baseball and football. The javelin action is not the usual throwing motion. To do it properly you have to use your body, generating all your power from your legs. I laugh when I see people pick up the javelin and the first thing they say is, "This is so light." Yeah, it's light, but I just smile and say, "Let's see you make it fly."

To learn the javelin I had to abandon everything I had learned about the throwing motion. Now, when I'm playing outfield for softball, I'll throw the ball to home plate and throw it right over the backstop. Why? Because I'm throwing with a javelin motion. It's not like baseball, where the elbow is the lead. In the javelin, you hold everything back until your left side clears, then your right side follows through. It requires an enormous amount of flexibility in the shoulder you're throwing with.

The javelin is an intensity sport: The more aggression you put into it, the more distance you're going to get. Small guys can throw the javelin well because it's all technique. It's about technique and explosiveness.

My best javelin performance was at the 1996 Olympics. It was intense, and my technique was right on. My worst experience was at the 1990 Goodwill Games when I only threw 190, and Dave Johnson threw 230 to catch up with me and win the gold.

The javelin is unique in the decathlon because it's the one event that isn't entirely natural. It's from the legs and the shoulder turn, and has little to do with the throwing action of the arm. If you throw too much you can hurt yourself. Because I don't want to hurt my legs or back, I'll take easy throws two times a week and throw hard only once every three weeks. It seems that every top javelin thrower I've ever met has had a shoulder operation, and I'm working at avoiding joining that group. I perform several stretches unique to the javelin and I do them just before a javelin practice. I also work on rotator cuff exercises, and my intense and frequent stretching also helps keep me injury free.

I always enjoy the javelin in a competition. For a decathlete, the javelin means there is only one event to go. You're able to relax a bit and actually have fun.

▲ 1500 METERS

Also known as the metric mile, the actual distance of the 1500 is 119 yards and 21.6 inches shorter than a mile. Because four laps of a conventional track is a mile, the athletes in this event at most United States tracks will not finish and start in the same place.

Although the 1500-meter distance seemed destined to replace the mile, as all the other running events are in meters, the mile has such appeal that it has been kept in competition. We hear of the first four-minute mile by Roger Bannister of Great Britain in 1954, but how about the first 3:45 in the 1500, or breaking 3:30 in the 1500?

Two of the most popular men in the 1500 were from Great Britain: Sebastian Coe, who broke the world record in 1979 with 3:32.1, and Steve Ovett, who broke it three times, ending with a best of 3:30.77 in 1983. Ovett was a media anomaly, because he ignored requests for interviews, and tended to irritate his opponents by waving to the crowd as he came down the home stretch.

The most amazing man in this event is unquestionably Noureddine Morceli of Algeria. He has broken the world record twice, with a best of 3:27.37 in 1995, but also has broken world records in the mile, 2000 meters, and the 3000 meters. Because distance runners tend to peak when they are older and he is still under 30, he has a promising future.

The best athletes in this event are usually light. Morceli weighs only 137 pounds. Again, for the decathlete, compromises must be made. In contrast to most 1500 meter runners, who stay at a steady pace throughout, decathletes have more fast-twitch fibers and as a result tend to have good kicks, making for many exciting finishes.

The 1500 is another event I've been doing only since I started competing in the decathlon. The 1500 is the only event that almost made me not do the decathlon. It's not fun. It's ten guys running on empty gas tanks. You just want it over with. I'm looking forward to it now, more than in the past. One interesting 1500-meter race occurred at the 1984 Olympic Games, when gold medalist Daley Thompson decided to jog the last lap of this event because he was so far ahead on points—even though a time near his best would have broken his own world record.

As a young athlete, I went out and just ran the 1500 hard. When you do that it hurts, and the memory of that pain sticks with me and still stands between me and a love for the 1500. Only a few decathletes ever look forward to the 1500 and are really good at it—Bruce Jenner was one. That was his event, and he looked forward to it because you look forward to what you're good at.

Because I'm outspoken about my dislike for the 1500, many people believe it's my worst event. That's not really true. I haven't run a bad 1500 in the last two years. I do nine things great, and one average. That's the 1500.

My best 1500 came in 1989 when I was running for eight thousand points, my personal best. I took off and ran with a guy who was a lot faster than I was, but I just kept going. It took ten minutes for me to recover afterward.

The only time I regretted not running faster in the 1500 was at the Goodwill Games in 1994 in Russia when I had a chance to break the record. Unfortunately, there were a lot of things going against me at the time. I was in Russia and there was nobody in the stands. I didn't want to be there in the first place, I knew I had the points to sew it up, and rather than thinking about record breaking, all I thought about was finishing the race and going home. I didn't know the event was on national TV, and a lot of the commentators hammered me afterwards, saying I didn't have the heart of a champion. But the fact is, we all have times like that; it's just that the cameras aren't usually on us.

I've had to work hard to like the 1500. To do that, I put in a lot of over-mileage. Right now I run five miles twice a week. This helps to make the one mile of the 1500 seem small in comparison. I'll even run a 5K from time to time. Why? Just to do it, to challenge myself a little bit more.

I work on my pace a lot, understanding seventy-second laps. Distance running is different from sprinting. You need to get a distance stride. It's hard for fast guys to find a stride they can hold for four or five minutes.

The 1500 is the end of the decathlon. For me, until I learn to have a love of this event, I remind myself that it's the end. I also realize that it's going to be all over in less than five minutes; and I know I can ask anything from my body if it's less than five minutes.

My goal in the decathlon is to set a record that will stand for five years, maybe ten. At Atlanta I penciled "9125" on my cap. Now that's a total that will stand, although I believe 9000, the goal I've written on a slip of paper in my pocket, will remain a goal. Why did I write "9125" on my cap? Because as an athlete you have to put your goals out there—way out there. You shoot for the best. When it comes to the 1500, I'm working at loving the event, and also running it as one of my best.

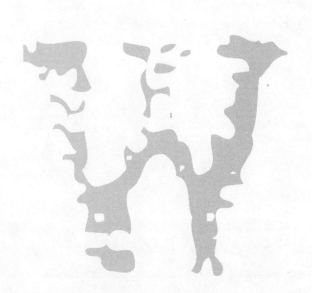

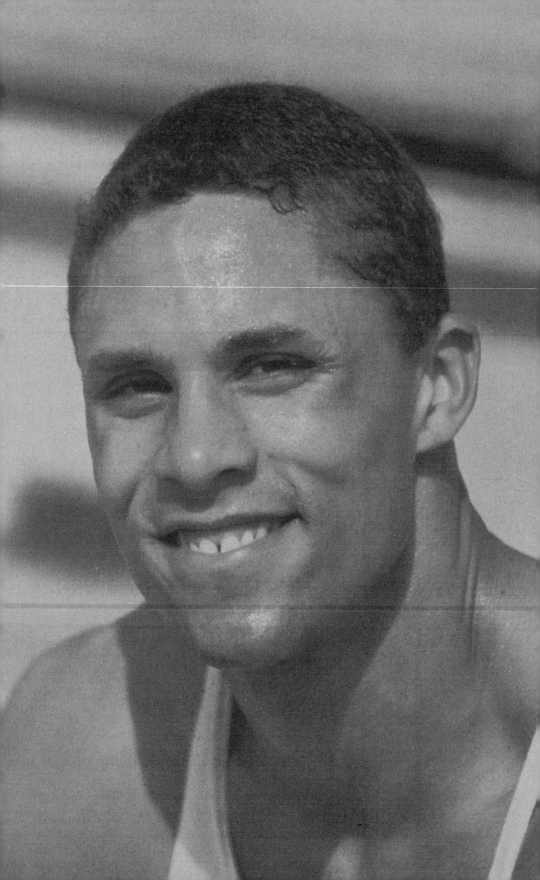

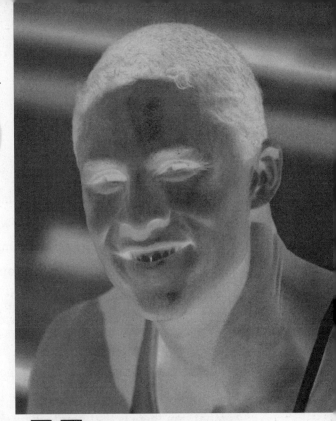

THE MOMENT
OF TRUTH

I n every competition there is a moment of truth, and it is in that moment that the winner and loser are determined. It may be the last meter, or the last seconds, or the last stretch, but one person succumbs and one person faces the moment of truth: To win, they must give their all. Every time I've faced this moment and given my all, I've come through.

At the Atlanta Olympics, my moment of truth came during the javelin. In 1995, it was the high jump. In every competition there is that point where you must, as Michael Johnson puts it, "slay the dragon."

The grueling nature of the decathlon has taught me that there is no substitute for hard work. An observer once said, "Whoever conceived of the decathlon was sadistic. They'd have to be to end the first day with the 400, then the second day, after nine events, with the 1500. That's downright cruel."

When I was in high school I didn't understand what it would take to be the World's Greatest Athlete. I didn't understand the hustle. I didn't understand that the more you can turn on, the more you can give. Today, I see this quality in athletes like Steve Young and Dan Marino. Watch their faces, and you'll see that the same concentration is etched in their brow and in the set of their jaw at the one-yard line or forty-yard line. They are focused and giving it all, whether the win is at hand or light-years away. That is what it takes to win.

Winners are athletes who continue to reach inside for more, to push on, to face the moment of truth, and conquer and quiet their greatest fears. They are the athletes who have discovered, channeled, and directed their energies to accomplish a single goal. They are the athletes who have learned that motivation is key to all accomplishments and is the fire that lights the way.

▲ GOAL SETTING

In 1990, I attended a seminar given by Milt Campbell, the 1956 gold medal decathlon winner. He recalled how, when he'd left for the the Olympics that year, he had told his mom he would be coming home with the gold, or he'd come home in a box. At the time, he was the most dedicated athlete I'd ever met.

Milt looked at his audience and asked how many of us had goals. I looked around the room of other aspiring athletes and we were all nodding our heads in affirmation. Of course we all had goals! Then he asked how many of us wrote them down. Again, most of us had. Then he asked how many of us had our goals in our pockets, right then. None of us moved, but Milt reached in his pocket and pulled out *his* goals and told us he did this every day, and every day he made certain he did one thing to help him achieve his goals. Then he looked at us and said, "You guys are athletes, and you need to do ten things!"

After the seminar, I went up to Milt and told him I wanted to be a great athlete. Milt looked at me and reminded me that I was already a great athlete. Then he asked me again what it was I *really* wanted to be. I replied, "The World's Greatest Athlete."

That night I went home and wrote down on a piece of paper, "World's Greatest Athlete." On the other side I wrote "9000 points," the score I want to achieve in the decathlon. That piece of paper is in my pocket right now.

That was a turning point for me. I'd always been a fast runner, and I knew I had potential because people told me I did. But my approach was based on fun; sports were fun for me, and I played them. I hadn't yet learned to work at them.

I fell into the decathlon by default. I'd always seen myself as a long jumper or hurdler. I dabbled in the decathlon in high school. I even managed to win the high school national championships and set the highest score in the decathlon, but it wasn't a serious effort. My natural running ability made up for my lack of skill in other events. In junior college in 1988, I decided to do the decathlon again, but I pulled a hamstring. Rather than compete at the championships, I was forced to sit on the sidelines and watch. What I saw didn't impress me. I knew I was faster—far faster—than the decathletes on the field. I knew then that I could learn the other events and turn my speed to its best advantage. So although the decathlon hadn't been my first choice, I saw an opportunity and went for it.

I realized that if I really wanted to become the World's Greatest Athlete, it would take more than an opportunity—it would take a lot of hard work. I realized that becoming the world's best at anything is a monumental task that necessitates hard work, dedication, and a precise plan.

Until then I was an average kid in college. I partied all night; I majored in fun. The parties interfered with my school, my grades fell, and I lost my scholarship. I was so embarrassed that I made up some excuse and told my mom I couldn't come home for Christmas. I woke up Christmas morning alone. Everyone else had gone home, and there I was by myself, with a garbage bag of empty beer cans propped up in the corner. I looked around and said, "This has to stop." That was it: one moment that changed the course of my life. I called my coach and said I wanted to get serious. He helped me get back into junior college and back on track, literally.

To accomplish anything, you first must have a vision—a goal. There should be no limits on that goal. Once you have a vision, then you need focus, persistence, discipline, and commitment. Those five words are extremely common in my vocabulary. I've lived by them. They are the principles that have made me successful.

I continue to work at applying those five principles in everything I do. I continue to check my goals each day and to do something every day toward accomplishing them. I've learned from Milt and other great motivational speakers. I've witnessed these five principles working for other people, among them Gail Devers, Pablo Morales, and Dan Jansen.

Athletes use a variety of mental crutches to enhance physical performance. Some jumpers won't go until they actually visualize their jumps in their minds. My mental crutch is an internal conversation. When I run, I'm always telling myself things: "Stay focused. Don't force it." I do it in all the events. In the hurdles, I tell myself to "ignore the people, pull ahead, now!" For the long jump it's "head up, head up, don't force the run." For me, these internal conversations keep me absolutely focused and in the event, always preparing for the next step.

To keep my motivation high, I've studied breathing techniques that help control the stress of competition. Working with different sports psychologists over the years, I've learned a technique of word association: I say a key word, then lie back and breathe slowly through the mouth. With enough practice you can learn to lower your heart rate in five to ten seconds. The same technique can be used to increase your adrenaline so that you're physically energized. These are techniques I'll practice driving in my car or at night when I go to bed.

In addition to breathing techniques, meditation tapes are great success builders. These tapes not only assist you in learning to use your breathing to control your mental and physical state, but they also help you reaffirm your goals and pinpoint your focus. I've also worked with psychologists over the years, not on sports performance, but on the core of Dan O'Brien. You have to make certain all aspects of your personality are straightened out in order to focus one hundred percent of your energy and abilities on the goal at hand.

It's absolutely essential for an elite athlete to learn to focus and prioritize. This is how I avoid distractions that can potentially come between me and my goals. When offers come up that will take me away from my training, away from my goal, I have to look at them carefully and weigh the benefit and the potential loss.

You also have to be ready to sacrifice. Being an athlete is about giving. Can you do another bench press? Can you make another run? How much can you sacrifice? During the past few years there have been times when I didn't visit or see my family for months. For years I didn't have a girlfriend. When you set a goal high enough, those are the kinds of sacrifices you have to make. Big goals require big sacrifices and absolute commitment.

I also took advantage of every motivational tool available. I knew that in order to make something happen on the track, it needed to happen in my mind first. I would get up in the morning and look at myself in the mirror and say, "Dan, you are the World's Greatest Athlete." That was when I began to act like an athlete, eat like an athlete, train like an athlete, and live like an athlete. When I came upon a challenging situation, I'd ask myself, "Is this something the World's Greatest Athlete would do?" When the answer was no, I avoided it.

Once I began to really focus on my goal, it became easier to expect greatness. Confidence in my abilities increased. Now, every time I step on the track, I know I'm going to win. Another great runner once commented that every time he ran, his mind was filled with doubt—doubt about who was going to come in second and third. That's the kind of mindset an athlete needs, and that was the mindset I began working with.

▲ World Records

I won't make any bones about the fact that winning the gold in Atlanta was one of the sweetest moments of my life. Winning again would be even sweeter. But until that happens, the greatest moment in my athletic career remains setting the world record.

World records drive athletes. Bruce Jenner touched on this, saying that going for a world record was a little like *Star Trek*—you're going where no one has gone before. It's hard to go into the unknown; it's scary. It was scary for me in France in 1992, particularly considering what had happened prior to the competition.

My no-heighter at the Olympic trials during the peak of the Reebok's multimillion-dollar "Dan and Dave" ad campaign stung. Except for actual competition, nothing can prepare you for the moment when they holler, "O'Brien up!" Your body and psyche are piqued, you're trying to maintain absolute control, and too often you tend to hold back. It gets easier with practice; but on that day at the 1992 Olympic trials, I was ill prepared. As a matter of fact, I hadn't pole vaulted all year long. Because of sponsorship commitments, I was giving speeches instead of practicing. I had forgotten my own rule to keep my training my number-one priority. The weather was hot and humid. Two other factors that may have contributed were a stress fracture I had earlier in the year and the fact that I had not competed outdoors leading up to the trials. Whatever the reasons, everyone knows the outcome: I no-heighted and lost my place on the 1992 Olympic team.

Bob Kersee called me at home that night. He told me not to try to prove anything, but just to get back into training. I didn't listen. Two weeks later I went to compete in Stockholm and had to pull out after three events. I went to the Barcelona Olympics as a commentator instead of an athlete, then I went home and went to work. I looked at all the things that had gone wrong at the trials. When I showed up in France, I was ready and I had a plan in place for any and every situation.

The weather was cloudy and cool, with a pretty good wind. Mostly the wind would be at our backs, giving us an advantage on the track. I'd had a great start in the first four events and had made personal bests in two of them, so I was feeling strong. The second day went equally well, and when I finally faced the pole vault, I had not only my no-heighter to deal with but also the fact that I was within three events of setting an impressive new world record. I'd already put the no-heighter behind me and was focused on the present. Now I needed to change that focus to a place somewhere ahead of me, to a world record, a place where no one had gone before!

I looked at the weather—it wasn't great. A headwind can make it difficult to get your tip down in the pole vault, and there was a bit of a headwind that day. I knew what I was up against; I had a plan for just such conditions. When they called "O'Brien up!" I was ready. I made it with room to spare, and from that moment on I was soaring. The javelin was like a blur, and the next thing I knew I was staring at the finish line of the 1500 with a new world record in the decathlon. I, Dan O'Brien, had totaled 8,891 points to set a new world record and, in that instant, had become the World's Greatest Athlete.

Still, no number of points could erase my no-heighter and my absence at the Barcelona Games from people's minds. I knew that I had to win the gold in 1996.

When I returned home, I focused on winning in Atlanta. There is no getting around the hard work, and work is what I did. At the 1996 trials, a big fuss surrounded my pole vault. What people didn't understand was that my no-heighter was a fluke and I'd put it behind me, I cleared a height of 17 feet, 3/4 inches, and despite less-than-par performances in the long jump and 1500 meters, I finished first on the United States team. I knew I would.

Atlanta, for me, was everything the Olympics should be for an athlete. I loved it. During the opening ceremonies I was with Michael Johnson, and we were both mobbed for pictures and autographs. A woman came up to us and asked if we'd like to get out of the mob scene and hang out with the dream team. It took us about a split second to say, "Okay, we can do that!"

I met all the basketball players and it was great. I was a little surprised that they didn't seem to care about the opening ceremonies. When we went down on the field, they stayed long enough for the cameras and were whisked away. They invited me to go with them but I wanted to stay. I didn't get home until two in the morning—I'd been walking around that field so long I had to get a calf massage the next day. I wouldn't have traded that night for anything.

I watched a lot of events, but for the most part, I practiced and stayed focused on why I was there. I wasn't there to win the bronze. I was there for one reason and one reason only: the gold. I thought back to Milt Campbell's pledge to his mom. I understood what he meant, and would have said the same thing to my mom, because I knew there was only going to be one outcome at the Atlanta Games.

Every event unfolded like clockwork. I floated over the hurdles; I soared in the jumps. I had done the work; I was there to collect the prize.

I won the gold in Atlanta and became "officially" recognized as the World's Greatest Athlete because I was prepared physically and mentally.

I still carry my goals on a piece of paper in my hip pocket. On one side is the goal I've accomplished: World's Greatest Athlete. On the other side is the goal I remain focused on: 9000 points. Of course, that second gold medal is going to look really nice next to the one I already have.

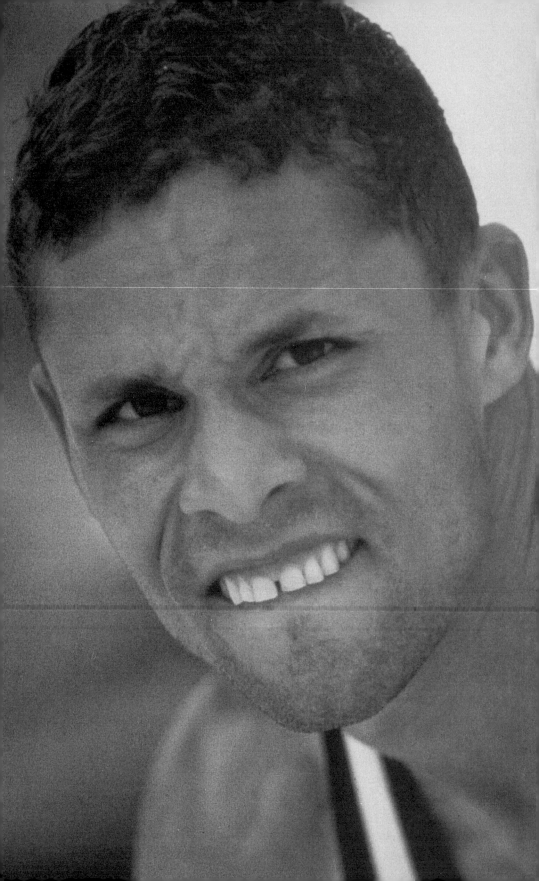

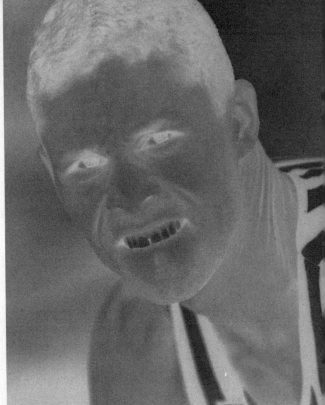

ELITE

ATHLETICISM

There's a responsibility that comes with being an athlete. One of the great things about being an athlete is the feeling that you are a part of history and tradition. When I stepped into the Olympic stadium in Atlanta, I knew I was part of something that went beyond just the challenge of the sport. And when I crossed the finish line of the 1500 meters, I was crossing it with Bob Mathias, Bill Toomey, and Bruce Jenner—I had joined the elite group of athletes who were considered the greatest in their era. My victory left me with not just a sense of accomplishment of achieving a goal, but also with an unforgettable sense of immortality. For the moment, for this era, I could rightfully call myself "The World's Greatest Athlete."

Because I love being an athlete and respect the traditions of sports, I have zero tolerance for the showboating and the swelled egos so prevalent in professional sports today. Having pride in one's accomplishments is one thing, but using one's success in athletics as a way to degrade others, to say, "I'm a better person than you," is not what sports should be about. Sports are a way to bring people together, to cross the boundaries of color and nationality. Sportsmanship extends far beyond the playing field—it's a way of conducting ourselves not only in competition, but also throughout our lives.

Participating in sports can play a major role in improving a person's attitude and ambition. My athletic career certainly helped me make some personal decisions that have positively altered my life. One of my most important choices was in college, when I was staying out late and drinking far too much beer. I don't believe I was an exception—on the contrary, I believe my partying was typical of a college jock. It would have been simple to fail, but instead, I took the hard road and strove to succeed. In addition, without belittling my own strengths and fortitude, I know I wouldn't be where I am today without the support of family, friends, and coaches.

This is a book about athletic achievement—yours and mine. Getting ourselves to that goal goes beyond the reps, sets, and drills we need to perform. It also has to do with attitude, motivation, determination, and dedication—the elements that define elite athletes and separate them from the mediocre. These are all areas in my life that have been enriched by other people who have provided advice, instruction, and role models to follow. To be a great athlete, you need to surround yourself with great people.

For an athlete it is essential to have heroes. I have literally hundreds of heroes from sports, movies, and myth. You need to find the heroes in your life, the men and women you want to emulate, the individuals whose standards you want to live up to. As an athlete, you'll find your heroes include a special group of individuals: your coaches.

Some of the high-profile sports, like gymnastics and figure skating, rely on a network of expensive, private coaches. That's not so with most track and field sports. The best place for a track-and-field athlete is school. In the United States, young athletes receive excellent coaching in track and field from high school right through the university system. And even though sports may be the only thing on your mind now, the education you get along the way will be a great asset you can use everywhere.

I can honestly say that I owe my career to my coaches. Over the years, there was something positive I learned from every one of them. Coach Sloan is without question the greatest decathlon coach I have ever worked with. He's helped me improve my skills in every event, while also teaching me the fundamental mindset to help me step into his shoes and become my own coach.

Coach Sloan's role in my achievements is great. And it is not only the sports skills that I'm referring to. A good coach goes beyond the playing field and teaches a person to be an athlete at heart.

▲ WINNING AND LOSING

Sports are competitions, whether against yourself, an opponent, or a team. Winning is the object of the game. But if an athlete has a winning-is-everything attitude, he or she may lose track of the spirit of sport, which is, in essence, play. After all, even at the Olympic level we *play* sports (albeit, under an intense pressure).

A good coach will help you discover this fine line between the winning-is-everything and sports-are-for-fun attitudes.

Coach Sloan often reminds me, "Winning isn't the only thing, but it sure is a lot of fun." Remember that as you try to win, strive to be the best you can be in all aspects as they pertain to the game. Also, appreciate the fact that for every winner, there must be a loser. The loser also puts forth his best effort, and a true athlete must appreciate that all-out effort given by another athlete because without it, his own accomplishment is diminished. A great athlete will show appreciation for another athlete's performance, whether it is a win or a loss.

Like all competitions, the decathlon is about winning and losing, but it is unique in the sense that an athlete can lose every event that he competes in and still win the overall competition. If I were to add ten feet to my personal best in the javelin but still place second to another athlete who threw a few feet further, would I be considered a loser? Perhaps to some people, but not to me. I would be thrilled, and would certainly take that performance over a lesser throw and first place in my event. My sense of accomplishment comes from knowing I've done my best, not recognition that I've beaten someone else.

Another valuable lesson a good coach will teach you is that winning is always a combination of elements: hard work, dedication, practice, talent, and circumstances. The first three can be controlled, the last two are largely twists of fate. When you win, you win not entirely of your own volition. Dan Jansen felt this when he won his gold medal in speed skating, and his gratitude was obvious to the world. I felt this as well when I received the gold. Many athletes show humility and thankfulness when winning because we've learned that, in spite of all the effort we put forth, part of the final outcome is directed by forces outside our control.

As important as it is to learn to win with grace, an athlete must also learn to lose with a healthy attitude. My no-heighter in 1992 was the perfect example. That performance could have marked the end of my career. Yet like the elusive win, a defeat is also the result of certain circumstances. You take stock of the situation, go back and make a new plan, and emerge again on the playing field better prepared. And along the way, you appreciate and congratulate those athletes who have enjoyed the winner's circle.

▲ WHAT A COACH WILL TEACH YOU

Many athletes play down the influence of their coaches upon their victories. Yes, as an accomplished athlete—a winning athlete—you have mastered the ability to be your own coach. But that doesn't lessen the role these mentors play in every athlete's development.

Many people ask me how they can shave a critical second off their time, add a foot to their jumping distance. The answer lies in finding proper coaching. A winning athlete needs to continually seek new training methods, attitudes, and approaches. Since we need to be on the practice field rather than in a library reading up on the latest Russian plyometric drill, we leave the job of finding those training innovations to our coaches.

Listen to your coaches—never try to do their job. Keep your mind open and always continue to seek. Just as in life you will have many influences, as an athlete you will have many coaches. Learn something from each of them.

▲ PUTTING IT ALL TOGETHER

This book has covered a lot of ground, from general fitness to the individual nuances of elite athletes. Let me leave you with a review of some of the major premises of my training program.

FLEXIBILITY:

I know that most up-and-coming athletes are more interested in how fast they can run and how far they can throw, but flexibility is a major factor in performance and longevity in any sport. So, while my program is far more extensive than the average person requires, it offers something for everyone.

If you are an aspiring track-and-field athlete, I cannot overstress the importance of beginning and maintaining a regular flexibility program. If you are trying to improve your sports performance, flexibility is one of the first areas you should work on—not that it will make a dramatic impact on your performance, but it will definitely prepare your body for the tougher training that is yet to come. If you are an older athlete in your thirties or forties, flexibility is an absolute must to maintain your range of motion and keep you injury free. Lastly, if you are a competitive athlete, you need to regard flexibility as a main component of your workout regimen.

STRENGTH TRAINING:

Many track and field books leave out the essential component of strength training, specifically, the application of weightlifting to track and field. Weightlifting is the ultimate crosstraining activity. It allows you to build complementary strength to assist you in your primary sport. More important, it enables you to avoid the muscle imbalances that plague so many athletes and that ultimately lead to injury.

One of the great features of my weight training routine is that it is useful in nearly all areas of life. My decathlon training requires such a wide range of strengths and skills that my weight training routine is one that will work for beginners, intermediates, track athletes, strength athletes, and power athletes, old and young. It is a very basic routine that anyone can use and benefit from.

BALLISTIC STRENGTH:

For many years, ballistic strength was considered to be a God-given talent of athletes blessed with a high ratio of fast-twitch muscle. Today's biomechanical sciences have come up with precise training protocols to enhance an athlete's ability to sprint, jump, and rotate. The benefits of this training component are obvious to the athlete; however, I feel it is equally important to the nonathlete in all of us. Developing ballistic strength puts a spring in your step and energy into your movements. Whether your sport of choice is tennis, golf, or volleyball, working on the drills I have shared in this book will increase your vitality as well as your physical performance.

ENERGY SYSTEMS:

Attention to your energy system, or cardiovascular training, is a fourth essential factor in sports performance. Athletes must know that their energy reserves from cardio training will be there when they push to their limits. However, the key to optimal endurance training is balance, as too much emphasis on aerobic system training can affect your speed and strength.

Those are the four components of my ultimate workout. Achieving optimum performance and good health involves applying smart exercise principles and something more: It takes motivation, incentive, desire, dedication, and good coaching. It has been my goal to inspire some of you to take more than a passing interest in the decathlon. For some, that may be actual competition; for others, it may mean you seek out an ESPN broadcast of a track-and-field event.

I've shared some of my greatest moments on the playing field, and also some of my insights into the techniques used by great athletes in each of the events. I've shared with you some of the early inspirations that helped me plot my career. When that moment of truth hits you, there are many ways the final decision can go. Planning every one of those possible scenarios—practicing them in my mind and on the training field—has helped me to win when it counts. As Coach Sloan says, "The will to win is nothing without the will to prepare." Whether your goal is in sports or in other successful and healthy life choices, the same principles apply:

1. You must have vision: a goal, a height to reach, an ambition to achieve.

2. You need focus: a clear and single-minded, task-oriented mindset.

3. You must work at it with persistence. Success rarely happens overnight, but often happens with a persistent effort. You have to stick with your plan.

4. Almost all success comes with a sacrifice, whether it's of time, lesser interests, or social life. You must accept that fulfilling a plan for success is going to require discipline on your part and the ability to let some things go to accomplish the larger goal.

5. Lastly, you need commitment. How hard are you willing to work? How badly do you want to achieve your goal? If you can say one hundred percent to both of these questions, then you have the commitment to accomplish whatever it is you desire.

Look for these other exciting products from Dan O'Brien:

Artwork by Jim O'Brien

1-800-282-5005

email: art2know@aol.com

Nutritional products by Cell Tech

1-800-800-9009

email: celltech.com

Reach me at my new Internet site

danobrien.com